Simplifying Eye Care

Dr. Quresh Maskati

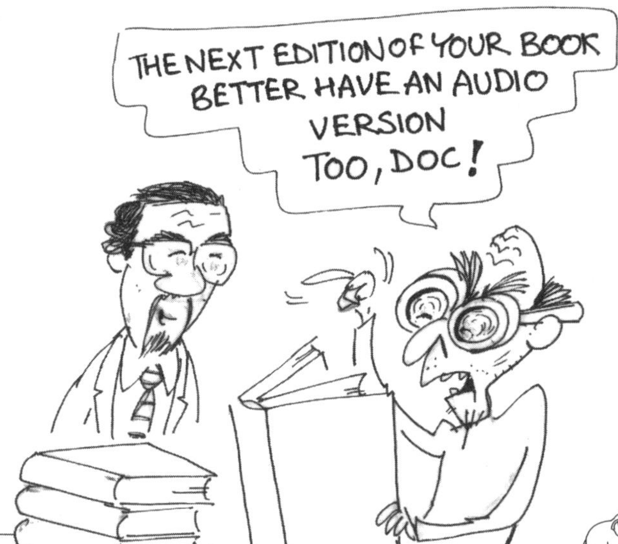

Popular Prakashan
www.popularprakashan.com

POPULAR PRAKASHAN PVT. LTD.
301, Mahalaxmi Chambers
22, Bhulabhai Desai Road
Mumbai 400026

ISBN 978-81-7991-597-4
(4345)

Design: Mahendra Ghanekar & Namita Jadhav
Illustrations: Hemant Morparia

Printed by
G. H. Prints Pvt. Ltd.
A 256, Okhla Phase I
New Delhi - 110 020

Published by Ramdas Bhatkal for
Popular Prakashan Pvt. Ltd.
301, Mahalaxmi Chambers
22, Bhulabhai Desai Road
Mumbai 400026

Dedication

To my patients, who have taught me more about ophthalmology and human psychology than anything I picked up in medical school. It was their persistent and intelligent questioning and their desire to know more about their ailments minus the technical jargon that inspired me to write this book…

FOREWORD

It is a novel idea to have a book which tells you about eye ailments in a simple and easy way. Whenever someone close to you undergoes treatment for an eye problem, there are many questions in your mind such as: What is the disease? How did it happen? How will it be cured and how long will it last? The answers to all these queries lie in this book.

Often the treating surgeon/clinician doesn't have enough time to talk to the patient in detail about the ailment and sometimes the explanation is not adequate or simple enough. This book is a handy tool in these situations.

I don't want to belittle the communication skills of my ophthalmologist colleagues, but it is difficult to explain complicated medical terms to a lay patient. This creates a barrier to fully understanding a disease and its management.

This is why I am sure this book will be useful for patients, their caregivers and to some extent, for general physicians and general ophthalmologists as well.

Prof. Rajvardhan Azad
MD (Ophth.) FRCS, FICS, FAMS
President, All India Ophthalmological Society
Professor of Ophthalmology
Chief, ROP & Vitreo-Retinal Services
Dr. R. P. Centre for Ophthalmic Sciences
All India Institute of Medical Sciences
New Delhi.

About The Author

Dr. Quresh Maskati has had a long and distinguished career as an ophthalmologist. He graduated from KEM Hospital, Bombay University. In 1983, he obtained his M.S., D.O.M.S & F.C.P.S. degrees, with a gold medal in DOMS. He has also obtained a super-specialisation in corneal diseases and anterior segment microsurgery from Rochester and Boston, USA.

Dr.Maskati is the only ophthalmologist in Asia to have done the Pintucci Keratoprosthesis on over 75 patients since 1997 and the only one in the world who has performed both the Dohlman Keratoprosthesis and the Pintucci Keratoprosthesis. He has also demonstrated Pintucci live in a number of South Asian cities including Kuala Lumpur, Manila and Karachi, besides various cities in India. He was awarded a gold medal for his pioneering work by the Indian Implant and Refractive Society in July 2007.

He has taken part in and conducted numerous camps for cataract and squint surgeries all over Maharashtra, Gujarat, Rajasthan and Madhya Pradesh since 1980 and has performed refractive surgery since 1998 - PRK, PTK, LASIK and currently, Wave-Front Guided LASIK.

He was ophthalmic advisor to Sight Savers International (formerly Royal Commonwealth Society for the Blind) for the whole of India, for six years, till 2004.

He has over two dozen scientific publications to his credit in national and international journals. He is co-author of chapters on Ophthalmology in nine books. He has devised and conducted an Ophthalmic Quiz at the National Conference every year, for 12 years.

He has the distinction of being the youngest person to hold the post of President of both the Maharashtra Ophthalmological Society (1994-95) and Bombay Ophthalmologists' Association (2000-01).

Dr. Maskati has been a guest speaker and visiting faculty at several international and national conferences.

Preface

I have wanted to write this book for a long time - a simple handbook on eye care that would help my patients. A book that would explain some common conditions that affect the eye and how best to prevent and treat them. There is a lot of information available today on the Internet, but not all of it is reliable or authentic. Most of the data is also hidden in mounds of unnecessary facts, so that it becomes difficult to separate the grain from the chaff. It is tough for an ordinary person to separate myth from fact.

I have tried to present information in as user-friendly a manner as possible. When writing it, I imagined that I was explaining a patient's condition to him in the simplest manner possible, in easy-to-understand terms. Wherever possible, I have talked about the preventive aspects of the disease or ailment.

For purposes of simplicity, I have, in most cases, referred to the patient in the masculine gender. I mean no disrespect to the by-far better gender!

I welcome comments from readers who found this book useful. I especially welcome critical comments so that I can make the next edition even more useful. If there are aspects which you feel I have ignored or tackled very superficially, do let me know so that I can include them or write about them in greater depth in future editions.

Please note that this small effort is in no way an exhaustive review of all aspects of and current knowledge in ophthalmology. In case you have any doubts or need any clarification about anything mentioned in the book, please consult your friendly neighbourhood ophthalmologist. Also, remember that every patient is unique and what applies to one patient may not necessarily be applicable to his friend, enemy, sibling, parent, cousin or municipal corporator!

I am sorry to put so many caveats in the preface itself. It is because a small section of the population has this nasty habit of quoting authors out of context and using patient guides such as these, to try and prove a point in every available (consumer) forum!

I think I have said enough – go ahead and enjoy the rest of the book!

Dr. Quresh Maskati

Contents

THE EYE

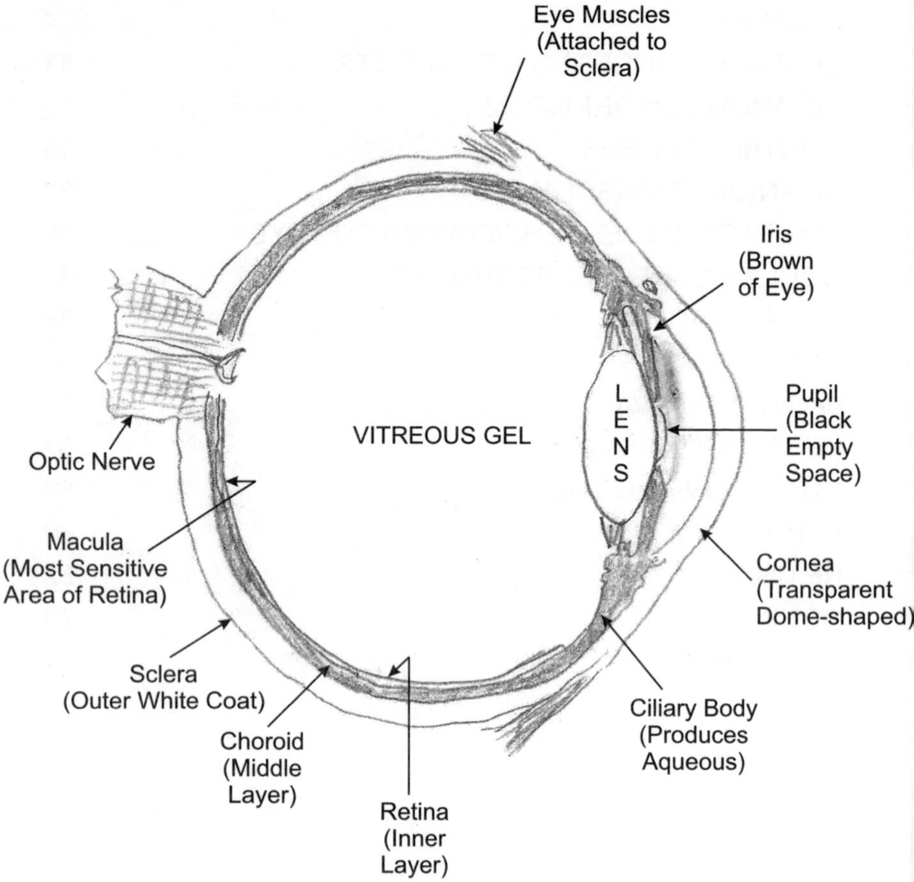
Eye Muscles (Attached to Sclera)
Iris (Brown of Eye)
Pupil (Black Empty Space)
LENS
VITREOUS GEL
Optic Nerve
Macula (Most Sensitive Area of Retina)
Cornea (Transparent Dome-shaped)
Sclera (Outer White Coat)
Ciliary Body (Produces Aqueous)
Choroid (Middle Layer)
Retina (Inner Layer)

Artificial Cornea or Keratoprosthesis (KP)

Kisan Jadhav (name changed) was studying for his master's degree in history in Jalna, a small town in central Maharashtra. He was a studious, quiet youngster, intent on realizing his dream of becoming a professor after completing his PhD. All that changed one day. Some miscreants, mistaking him for someone else, threw acid upon his face. He was admitted to the local hospital with extensive facial chemical burns and both eyes severely damaged.

Several painful reconstructive surgeries later, his face regained some semblance of normalcy. But he was totally blind in both eyes. The left eye had shrunk to a third of its size and could not even perceive light. Though the right eye could perceive light, the cornea was totally opaque and the eye was bone dry. With virtually no tear production, a corneal graft was doomed to fail.

Fortunately, his eye surgeons had heard of a new treatment suitable for such patients. He was referred to Mumbai and operated upon in two stages and an artificial cornea or Pintucci Keratoprosthesis was implanted in his right eye. It is now one year since this surgery. Kisan has 6/6 or normal distance vision with glasses and can read the tiniest of print without any glasses. He has resumed his studies and has passed his MA exam.

Q. Who is a suitable candidate for KP?

A. A patient who is blind in both eyes but at least has accurate perception of light in the better eye can undergo KP surgery, which can be done in only one eye. A patient with an opaque cornea who has been refused corneal transplant because of dry eye, much vascularised cornea, diseases like pemphigus or Stevens Johnson syndrome or chemical burns where corneal transplant is not advisable, can be a candidate for the surgery.

Q. I have had multiple failed corneal grafting surgeries. Can I be operated for KP?

A. Yes, provided a sonography shows that your retina is intact and there is no severe glaucoma.

Q. Is this surgery expensive?

A. Yes. The Pintucci Keratoprosthesis, which is imported from Europe, is very costly. Besides, the surgery is technically demanding, done in two stages, two months apart. Surgery in each stage lasts for 2-3 hours and is generally done under general anaesthesia. Some tissue is also taken from the patient's mouth. It is however cheaper than a cochlear implant for hearing restoration or cardiac surgery.

Q. Can this surgery be a substitute for corneal graft?

A. No. This surgery should be considered as a last resort only. It is done only for those who have failed grafts or in whom grafting is not advisable. Corneal grafting is still the first treatment of choice for those with opaque corneas and adequate tears.

Q. Can the KP be rejected?

A. No. It is made of the same material that most IOLs (Intra-Ocular Lenses) are made of — polymethylmethacylate or PMMA, which is an inert plastic.

Q. What is the success rate?

A. The author has operated on approximately 75 patients so far, with a follow-up of 12 years. The success rate i.e. patients retaining useful vision after the surgery is 65%. The late Dr. Stefano Pintucci, the inventor of this device, had handled over 1500 cases over 20 years with a similar success rate.

Q. Are there other KP devices?

A. The three commonest designs available in the market besides the Pintucci are:

- The Daljit Singh champagne cork KP. It uses stainless steel sutures to secure the KP in the eye. It is the largest series reported in the world.
- The OOKP or Osteo-Odonto KP also called the "eye-in tooth" KP. The surgery can be done only in adults by a team including a dentist as it requires use of a healthy canine tooth from the patient. Besides Rome, Italy, it is done in Birmingham, UK and in Singapore in significant numbers. In India, a few have been implanted, mainly in Chennai.

- The Boston KP or the Dohlman KP. This is an American design, which is very popular in USA and Latin America. It is a simpler technique that is done in one stage and requires a donor cornea. The cosmetic appearance is also better.

The author has done this procedure in Mumbai since February 2009, in select cases. He has also demonstrated this surgery to an audience of 200 ophthalmologists in Bangalore, restoring sight to a man blind in both eyes for over a dozen years prior to the surgery.

Q. Is there a difference in patient selection criteria for the Pintucci and the Boston KP?

A. Yes. For Boston KP, the patient needs to have some amount of tear production. He should not have any history of corneal melt, nor should he suffer from systemic diseases that could result in corneal melt. Therefore it is done in damaged or diseased corneas where the disease is less severe. For very severe dry eyes, with melted corneas such as in Stevens' Johnson Syndrome or chemical injuries, the Pintucci KP works best.

Cataract

Q. What is a cataract and how is it formed?

A. Any opacification of the human lens of the eye is called a cataract. The human eye is like a camera – the front portion, which is clear and transparent, is called the cornea. The lens is biconvex, exactly like the lens of a conventional camera and is situated behind the pupil of the eye (the jet-black window in the brown/blue/green iris of the eye). It is made up of protein and water and is normally transparent. Due to the aging process, these lens proteins coagulate, losing their transparency over time. Certain drugs such as steroids as well as certain diseases such as diabetes hasten this biochemical change. Several studies blame pollution, cigarette smoking and prolonged exposure to the ultraviolet rays of the sun as some causative factors. The reason it occurs in some people at 45 while others live to be a 100 without developing any cataract is at present unclear. Whenever we doctors cannot give a logical explanation, we normally say there must be a genetic factor either causing the development of cataract or preventing it in different sets of patients.

Q. Is there a medical treatment for cataract?

A. Unfortunately (for patients – fortunately for eye doctors!) there is no scientifically proven medical treatment for cataract. There are plenty of grandmother's remedies touted as cures or preventive treatments, such as honey, certain vegetable extracts, cow's urine and even auto-urine therapy. None of them work. There are also a host of eye drops made by homoeopathic and ayurvedic companies which burn and sting on application (besides burning quite a hole in the pocket!), which claim to stop the progress of cataract. None of them work. The reason they become popular is that many a time the cataract can stop progressing or remain stationary for years on its own, for reasons which are unknown. If at that time the patient is using any of the above remedies, he will tell a minimum of 50 people about the miraculous drug or therapy, convinced that that is the reason for the lack of progress of the cataract. Usually, patients who are not undergoing therapy and in whom the cataract has not progressed are not known to brag!

Q. Does every cataract patient need to undergo surgery?

A. Just as every one does not have to climb Mount Everest just because it is there, so also you do not have to undergo cataract surgery just because your doctor has diagnosed that you have a cataract. You will need to undergo surgery only if the cataract has progressed to such an extent that it hampers your day-to-day activities. This varies tremendously from person to person. A 50-year-old executive may feel handicapped if he finds it difficult to read the fine print on important contracts that he has to sign daily. On the other hand, a 75-year-old housewife with a more advanced cataract may have no complaints if she is still able to read the large print of her religious books! The executive may require surgery for his early cataract while I may ask the housewife to see me after a year for reassessment.

Q. If I delay my cataract surgery, it may become too 'ripe' or may 'burst' and I may lose the eye permanently. Is that true?

A. Not true. A cataract is considered 'over-mature' or in danger of rupture only if it is pearly white in appearance or if the vision has deteriorated so much that the patient can only see light projected into his eye but cannot recognize objects even from a distance of

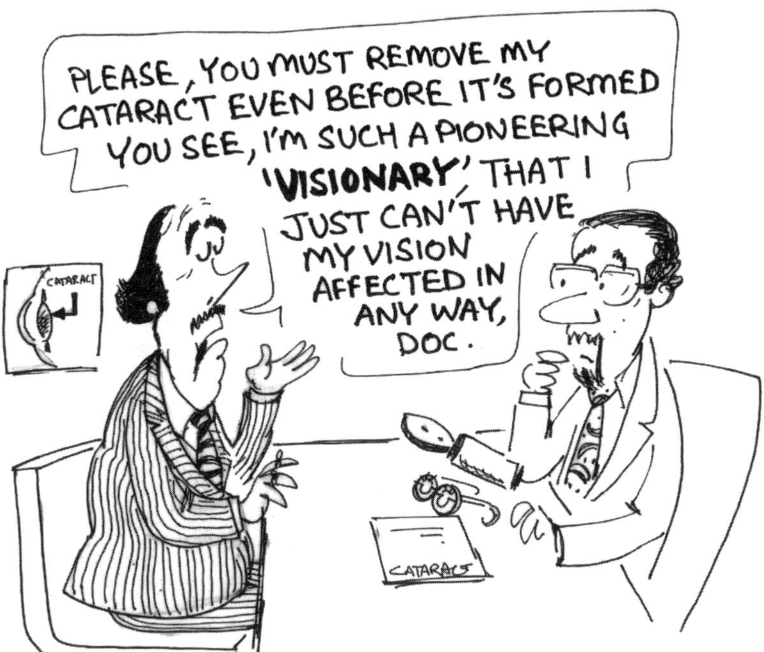
PLEASE, YOU MUST REMOVE MY CATARACT EVEN BEFORE IT'S FORMED YOU SEE, I'M SUCH A PIONEERING 'VISIONARY' THAT I JUST CAN'T HAVE MY VISION AFFECTED IN ANY WAY, DOC.
CATARACT
CATARACT

less than one metre. As long as you go for regular check-ups once in every six months or a year, your ophthalmologist will be able to recommend surgery long before that stage is reached.

Q. If I delay my surgery, will the cataract become too 'hard'?

A. It is true that brown and black cataracts may harden over time, making their surgery a little more difficult. However, with modern-day methods, they no longer pose a problem for an experienced eye surgeon.

Q. What is 'phacoemulsification'? Is it different from laser surgery?

A. Phacoemulsification is the use of a machine to which a pencil-like probe is attached. It vibrates at a very high frequency emitting ultrasonic energy. This breaks up or emulsifies the lens ('phakos' is Greek for 'lens') into tiny bits, which are then sucked out through tiny openings in the probe. This is what the lay public refers to as 'laser surgery'. In fact, laser is not used at all in these machines. 'Laser cataract surgery' is simply a myth. Probably a few black sheep in the ophthalmic fraternity who do not have the time to explain Phacoemulsification to their patients, or who feel their patients' I.Q. level will not allow them to understand such big words, combined with some inaccurate and exaggerated stories in the press, have helped spread the myth of 'laser cataract surgery'.

However, there are indeed a handful of genuine laser machines, which are used in combination with Phacoemulsification machines. But these machines take more time and cannot remove hard cataracts and therefore have proved very unpopular with most cataract surgeons.

Q. What are the other methods of cataract surgery?

A. While experienced surgeons can remove all cataracts using the phaco machine, others may also use non-phaco methods for certain types of cataracts such as very hard cataracts or very soft cataracts which are difficult to remove safely using the phaco machine. Surgeons employing non-phaco methods may use a small sutureless incision to enter the eye, or a larger incision which will need to be closed with stitches.

Q. Is any method superior to the others?

A. That is a loaded question! Phacoemulsification and the small incision non-phaco method are both 'sutureless'. Hence the patient heals faster. Usually the patient sees fairly well in about a week or so and can return to a normal life with no restrictions. A patient who undergoes a larger incision surgery with sutures may take four to six weeks to regain good vision. Some 'sutured' cases may have slightly higher 'astigmatism' or cylinder number left over at the end of six weeks as compared to the sutureless surgeries. However, in a majority of cases, there is almost no difference in the appearance of the eye or the best-corrected visual acuity at the end of six weeks, irrespective of the method used.

Q. How will I know which method is best suited to me?

A. If you trust your ophthalmologist, let him decide how he will extract the cataract from your eye. The procedure he will choose will depend on different factors e.g. the type of cataract you have, your lifestyle, his experience etc.

Q. What is an IOL (intra-ocular lens) implant?

A. The IOL is a thin plastic, acrylic or silicon lens. The first implants were used shortly after the Second World War, but complications arose. They were then modified and have since been in use from the early eighties. Today, almost all cataract surgeries in the world are done with the simultaneous implantation of IOL.

Q. Is the IOL safe? What is its lifespan?

A. It is extremely safe. As the material of the lens is biologically inert, it is not rejected by the body. Judging from the vast majority of successful surgeries over the past two decades, it can be said that there should be no problems due to the lens during the average lifespan of the patient.

Q. Are imported IOLs superior?

A. Patients are more than willing to buy an imported, but more expensive IOL. But I am proud to say that Indian IOLs have come of age and are even exported to over 50 countries in Europe and the Americas. They are as good as and in some cases even superior to their imported counterparts. However, as with most other gadgets and gizmos, there is the craze for foreign IOLs among the patients, which eye surgeons happily satisfy, as the patient does not mind paying a bit more for an imported IOL!

Q. What are rigid and foldable IOLs?

A. Rigid IOLs are lenses made of a medical grade plastic called PMMA and have a maximum width of 5 to 6 mm. They can be inserted after any type of cataract surgery by cutting an incision of approximately the same size in the eye.

The foldable IOLs made of acrylic or silicon material can be folded and slipped into the eye through an incision as small as 1mm. These can be inserted only after a cataract is removed by phacoemulsification. At present, yellow IOLs are the most expensive foldable IOLs available in the market. They are lenses coated with a special pigment to give the patient clearer vision, especially for night driving.

Efforts are on to mass-produce IOLs, which can be inserted through even smaller incisions. Smaller the incision, less is the chance for astigmatism or cylinder number.

Q. What are multifocal IOLs?

A. Multifocal IOLs are special IOLs, which can correct both distant and near vision thereby reducing the patient's dependence on glasses. They are a little more expensive than the other IOLs, but are not suitable for all candidates.

Q. Is general anaesthesia needed for surgery?

A. No. All you need is an injection of local anaesthetic around the eye. After the surgery, a patch is applied to keep the eye closed for few hours. The eye patch is not needed if the surgeon applies only topical drops of anaesthesia, with no injection. However, serious complications can arise if the patient inadvertently moves the eye or blinks hard during the surgery. It is best to discuss this aspect too with the surgeon before surgery, to prevent him from blaming you for any mishap later. Make sure, in case the surgeon is going to use only topical anaesthesia, that he is well experienced and is not doing this only to impress you! A tiny, tiny percentage of eye surgeons claim to operate on patients with no anaesthesia at all, not even topical drop anaesthesia. Thankfully, the tribe of such surgeons is not growing.

Q. How soon will I start to see clearly after the surgery? Will I need glasses after the surgery?

A. It depends on the type of surgery. If you have had surgery with topical anaesthesia, you will see reasonably well immediately after the surgery. If you have been patched, you will see reasonably well after the patch is removed.

Some eye surgeons leave an air bubble between the cornea and the implant for added safety. This air bubble can considerably blur the vision for up to a week post-surgery. If your surgeon has used sutures to close the incision, clarity may come only after a month or so. Most patients will develop a small number after the surgery and will need glasses to see clearly. Wait for four to six weeks after the surgery for the number to stabilize before having glasses made.

Q. What are the dos and don'ts after surgery?

A. These vary from case to case. The number of don'ts has dropped drastically over the years as cataract surgery has become safer. Most surgeons allow you to wet your head about a week after the procedure. In case of stitches, you may have to wait longer. There is usually no restriction in diet. Otherwise, you can read, write, watch TV, bicker with your spouse and shout at your kids almost immediately after the surgery.

Q. Do I have to stop the medications I take for other medical conditions?

A. Not always. Please inform your doctor if you are on aspirin for thinning the blood. He may ask you to stop these tablets a few days before and after the cataract surgery. If you are a diabetic, your anti-diabetic pills may have to be omitted on the morning of surgery.

Q. My vision was fine after the surgery. But it began to blur after six months. My doctor has advised 'YAG laser treatment'. What is it?

A. In some patients, the bag into which the IOL is inserted becomes opaque with time. This may happen as soon as one month after surgery, many years later or most probably not at all. This condition can occur even after a perfect surgery. It is not a complication of surgery but an unpredictable side-effect causing blurry vision. It can be corrected by a painless 5-minute procedure called "YAG laser capsulotomy" in which a laser beam is used to burn a small hole in the centre of the capsule to restore the patient's vision. This is a one-time procedure which does not usually have to be repeated.

Q. Can a person operated for cataract donate his eyes after death?

A. Most certainly! Though the whole eyeball of the donor is removed after death, only the transparent layer in the front of the eye called the cornea is used. As it normally remains unaffected by successful cataract surgery, the cornea can restore sight to another blind person through a successful cornea transplant.

Common Concerns of Parents

Q. When should I first take my child to see an eye doctor even if he has no apparent problem?

A. Ideally at 2.5 to 3 yrs of age and definitely before he turns 5. Problems like unequal spectacle number or a number only in one eye can be detected at a very young age and rectified. If the child has a problem only in one eye, a contact lens in that eye will prevent the development of a "lazy" eye.

Q. My child has not yet learnt to read the alphabet. Can her eyesight be checked?

A. Of course! A child does not necessarily need to know how to read to get her eyesight checked. The doctor does not need the cooperation of the child.

Q. What if my child does not want to wear spectacles?

A. It is often the parents' attitude which governs the child's like or dislike of spectacles. You should persuade your child to wear the prescribed glasses with love and patience. Don't force him to wear them constantly from day one. Let him get used to them gradually – let him try them on for 10 minutes on the first day, half an hour on the next day and so on.

Q. Can I opt for laser surgery for my child?

A. No. Excimer laser surgery to correct spectacle number is not recommended till the patient is at least 18 years of age and the number has stabilised i.e. it has not increased in the past one year.

Q. My five-year-old son has a plus five number. Will it increase with age?

A. No. Normally, as the child grows up, the eyeball also grows in size. So, plus numbers have a tendency to decrease with age.

Q. My daughter wears a minus 5 number. Are her eyes 'weak'?

A. No. Minus numbers occur in a condition known as 'myopia' or short sight. This means that the child can see nearby objects well but has problems seeing distant objects. This occurs when the cornea and the lens bend the rays of light so much that they focus the image in front of the retina. It does not mean that her eyes are 'weak'.

Q. Will the minus number reduce over time?

A. As the eyeball grows, the retina moves further back in relation to the cornea and lens. Hence it is likely that a minus number may increase with time.

Q. Can the number be prevented from increasing?

A. There is no medically proven method to prevent the number from increasing, including the use of contact lenses. In fact this is like making your child wear a hard hat over his head to prevent the height from increasing! However, it is a fact that numbers, like height, are genetically pre-determined and so a child's minus number could stop increasing suddenly at say age 12 or 14. If at that time, the child was doing natural exercises, or wearing a contact lens, or putting honey in the eyes, or even practising urine therapy, that particular treatment is given wide publicity by gullible parents. This results in neighbours, friends and relatives insisting

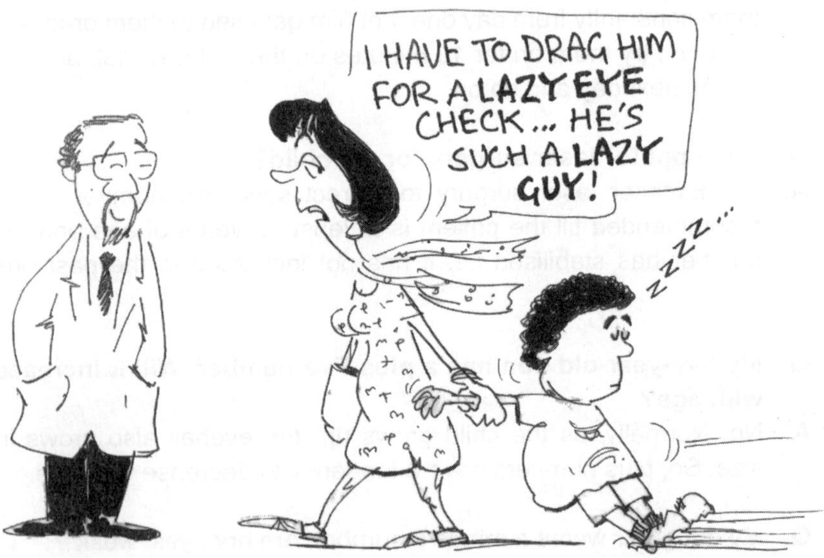
I HAVE TO DRAG HIM FOR A LAZY EYE CHECK... HE'S SUCH A LAZY GUY!
ZZZZ...

that this or that therapy is incredibly successful in preventing increase in numbers!

Q. Do wrong reading habits or watching too much TV cause an increase in numbers?

A. Generally, minus numbers are genetically pre-determined and their increase cannot be controlled. In an interesting study done in Japan, children from similar genetic stock were divided into 2 groups. One group studied only in English for 10 years while the other studied only in the complicated Japanese script. At the end of the 10-year period, more students studying Japanese ended up wearing minus-numbered glasses. Therefore, there may be an environmental factor contributing to increasing numbers. However, there is no unanimity on this subject.

Q. Should my child avoid physical activity or contact sports if he has a minus number?

A. Not at all. Most short-sighted children tend to prefer indoor activities and books to outdoor sports. However, you should encourage your child to take up physical activity and explore the world outside with his glasses on.

Q. My child has a 'high' minus number. Will he suffer from problems later?

A. It is true that myopes are more prone to retinal detachment. However, an annual retinal examination by your eye doctor will reveal any thinned out areas of the retina that may require preventive treatment. If none exist, your child can have a normal life without restrictions despite his 'high' minus number.

Q. Will a child with 'shaking eyes' go blind with time?

A. No. 'Shaking eyes' or nystagmus as it is called, is a to-and-fro searching movement of the eyes. It occurs when the central portion of the retina, which controls fine vision, is not fully developed. This is common in albinos (children who lack skin pigmentation). In most conditions, the vision usually improves with time and the nystagmus decreases in severity over the years.

Q. How often should I take my child to the eye doctor for a check-up?

A. If the change in numbers is slow and steady, once a year may be sufficient. However, if the child has visual complaints or headaches, it means the numbers have changed and the child may have to be taken for a check-up more often.

Q. Can I not have my child's eyes examined by an optician? After all, he does not charge me for the eye examination!

A. Remember, an optician can only check for numbers – he is not qualified to examine the retina, which the eye doctor will do on every visit. Moreover, opticians rely on fancy "computerised" machines to prescribe glasses for children. These methods are inadequate and definitely not substitutes for the old-fashioned manual examination that eye doctors perform.

Common Concerns...2

Q. Is it all right to use honey or rose water to soothe tired eyes?

A. If your eyes feel tired, it is better to avoid infection by using simple sterile lubricant drops which are available over the counter without a prescription, instead of any home-made substances.

Q. Does walking on green grass with bare feet benefit the eyes?

A. There is no scientific basis for the belief that walking barefoot on green grass is good for the eyes. It is neither beneficial nor harmful for the eyes.

Q. Are 'palming', moving the eyes in all directions and other eye exercises helpful?

A. These exercises neither help to reduce the number of the spectacles, nor do they benefit the eyes in any way.

Q. What kind of diet is good for my child's eyes?

A. The normal Indian vegetarian diet with pulses, vegetables, *chapatis* and rice contains adequate amounts of Vitamin A for the growing child as do all non-vegetarian diets. If the child is a fussy eater, does not eat home-cooked food adequately or has only junk food, he will probably not have the right levels of Vitamin A in his body. In such cases, giving him two glasses of milk everyday is recommended. Be warned...too much of Vitamin A, such as daily doses of carrot juice, can actually harm the child – it can result in a higher incidence of sterility in males in adulthood!

Q. What precautions should I take to prevent my child from getting infected with 'sore eyes'?

A. Conjunctivitis (sore eyes) is highly contagious. Avoid sending your child into crowded areas like swimming pools. If a child displays the symptoms of sore eyes i.e. redness and discharge from the eyes, he should not attend school till the discharge subsides as he can infect others. If a sibling at home is infected, he should avoid

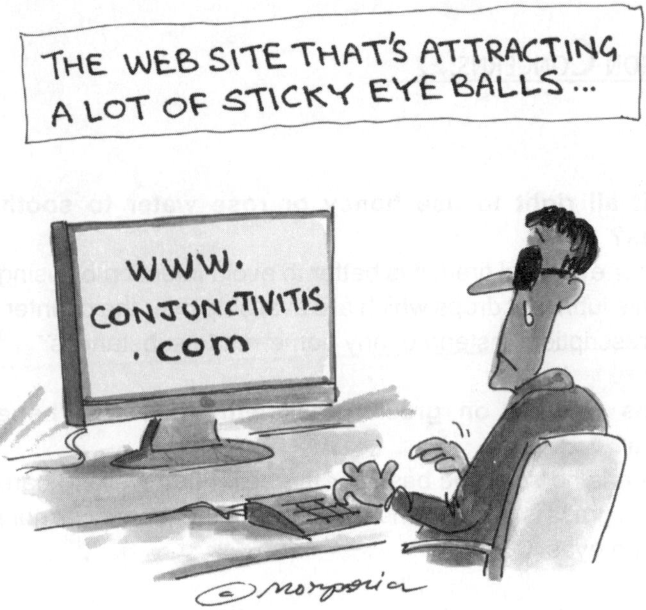
THE WEB SITE THAT'S ATTRACTING A LOT OF STICKY EYE BALLS...
WWW.
CONJUNCTIVITIS
.COM
©Morparia

physical contact with the sibling. An infected child should have his clothes, handkerchiefs etc. washed separately to avoid the spread of the infection.

Q. What can my child do to better protect his eyes?

A. Though the minus number is hereditary, observing correct visual habits can certainly help to reduce the strain on your child's eyes.

- ✦ He should always watch TV or read in the sitting posture, not lying down either on the stomach or the back.
- ✦ The child should view the TV or computer screen directly and not from an angle.
- ✦ Ensure that the child takes a break of 30 seconds to a minute every 30-45 minutes whenever he has to concentrate for long hours, while reading, or watching TV, or working on the computer. Simply staring out into the distance or gently shutting his eyes will give his eyes much-needed rest.
- ✦ He should read in a room with adequate light. Generally speaking bulbs are better for the eyes than tube lights. This does not mean that every parent should change the light fixtures in the room. Many children forget to switch on the

room lights at dusk, so engrossed are they in their reading. Reading in poor light causes a strain on the eyes. This should be avoided.

- Whenever the child has extra studying to be done, such as during examinations, it is better to wake up early and read when the eyes are fresh rather than read late into the night, when the eyes are already tired having been strained throughout the day. Grandmother's adage of "early to bed, early to rise" is excellent advice for kids appearing for exams.
- Children should avoid reading or playing video games in moving vehicles, such as cars, trains etc. Trying to concentrate, especially on a bumpy road, puts more strain on the eyes. Reading in an aeroplane is okay, of course!

CONTACT LENSES

Q. Most kids nowadays do not wish to wear glasses at all and usually prefer contact lenses. Is it ok?

A. No, it is not ok. All children with spectacle numbers should be encouraged to wear a pair of spectacles. However, older children, like those who are around 15 years of age, can wear, remove and maintain the contact lenses on their own without help. They may be allowed contact lenses at the discretion of the eye doctor.

Q. Is looking after contact lenses very difficult?

A. If you do not follow the doctor's instructions you can get your eyes into trouble. There are several dos and don'ts as far as contacts lenses are concerned:

- Contact lenses should never be worn for longer than 8 to 10 hours at a stretch.
- Most contact lenses should not be worn overnight.
- You should put on and remove the lenses with clean hands.
- The recommended cleaning/disinfecting solution should be used to clean and store the lenses and the carrying case.
- The case should be changed frequently.
- The lenses should be replaced as per the recommended schedule.
- The patient should report the first sign of trouble, e.g. a red eye, persistent watering, pain, blurred vision etc. to the eye doctor immediately.

  I am not trying to dissuade you from letting your child wear contact lenses, but patients have permanently lost their eyesight to severe infections just because they did not follow the prescribed hygiene strictly.

Q. What are the types of contact lenses available?

A. Traditionally, three types of contact lenses are manufactured - the hard or rigid lenses, the semi-soft or gas permeable rigid lenses and the soft lenses. However, most people today use the soft lenses. The hard and semi-soft are used for special indications, such as corneas with conical shapes (keratoconus), very high astigmatism (cylindrical numbers) or corneas scarred by previous injury or infection. People who are currently using hard or semi-soft lenses and are happy with them can continue wearing them. They are perfectly safe – you do not have to switch to soft lenses just because they are available!

Q. Are there many types of soft lenses?

A. Today, there is a lot of choice in soft lenses and I am not talking just of the various companies marketing them! The conventional soft lenses are the daily wear lenses (lenses that are removed and stored at night), which should be replaced ideally once a year or earlier if they give trouble. There are also the disposables — monthly, fortnightly, weekly and daily disposables.

Q. My teenage daughter wants to wear disposable lenses for a wedding. Are they safe?

A. Daily disposable lenses require less maintenance as they are thrown away before the proteins and other impurities get

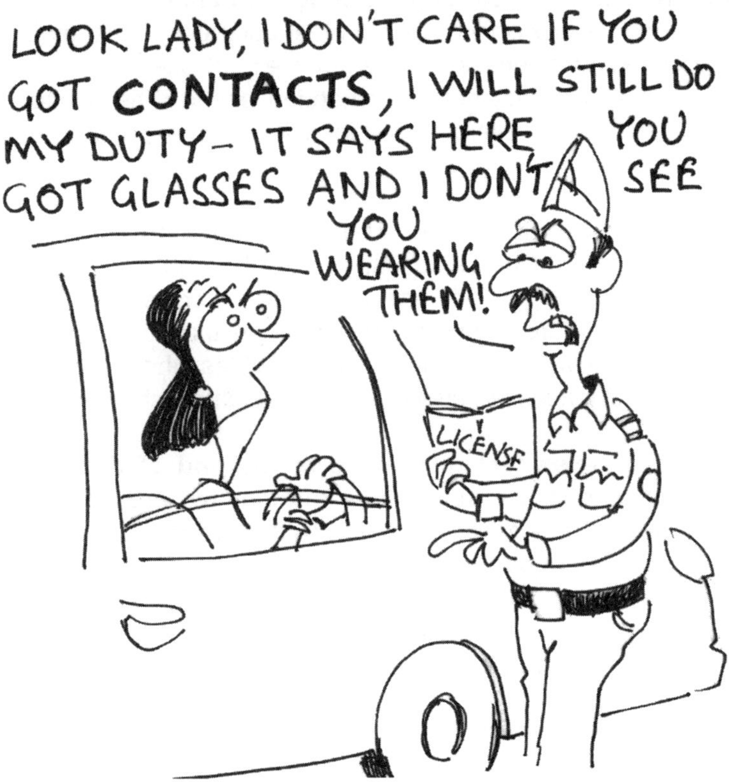
LOOK LADY, I DON'T CARE IF YOU GOT CONTACTS, I WILL STILL DO MY DUTY- IT SAYS HERE YOU GOT GLASSES AND I DON'T SEE YOU WEARING THEM!
LICENSE

permanently stuck to the surface. You simply open a sterile pack and throw away the lenses after the day/party is over! The greatest advantage of the daily disposables is doing away with the hassles of a lens case and cleaning solutions. It is a great cost-effective option if you are a regular spectacle wearer and wish to wear contact lenses only for social occasions like a wedding.

Q. Do monthly disposables have to be discarded after wearing them on 30 occasions or 30 days?

A. This is a mistake made by many patients. If you open a 30-day disposable lens pack, you must throw away the lenses 30 days after opening the pack. This is irrespective of whether you have worn them for only 10 days or 20 days or each of the 30 days after the pack was opened. The same holds true for fortnightly and weekly disposable lenses – they must be thrown away after a fortnight and a week respectively.

Q. I think you have been bribed by the lens manufacturing industry. My friend wears her monthly disposables for two months before discarding. Nothing happens!

A. Your friend is lucky. You may not be equally lucky. Most problems associated with lenses stem from their misuse. This includes using them beyond the recommended period. The chances of developing ocular allergies and infections rise exponentially with such misuse.

Q. Can I still wear soft lenses if I have astigmatism?

A. Yes. Astigmatism or cylindrical number is a 'focusing number'. Nowadays, you get 'toric' soft lenses which correct astigmatism as well. They are a little more expensive than the regular soft lenses. However, if the cylinder number is less than 0.75, regular soft contact lenses will also give you adequately sharp vision.

Q. Lately my eyes feel quite tired at the end of the day. My contact lenses are sometimes difficult to remove and the eyes feel a little sore, but I feel better when I splash some water into my eyes. There is a mild redness after I remove the lenses. Earlier, I could easily wear my lenses for 10-12 hours at a stretch, but now I feel like removing them after 6-8 hours. What is happening?

A. You are suffering from 'dry eye' induced by your contact lenses. This occurs in a small percentage of contact lens wearers even if they follow all the instructions given by the eye doctor. The contact lens causes our normal tear film to become a bit unstable; it promotes the evaporation of tears leading to mild 'dry eye'. This causes all the symptoms you have described.

This phenomenon is commoner in patients who misuse their lenses or are constantly glued to the small screen – TV, laptops and desktop computers. When you are engrossed in watching the screen, you inadvertently blink less, leading to inadequate spread of tears across the eye and greater evaporation from the ocular surface.

Q. Enough about the problem. What is the solution?

A. Firstly, try blinking more often when you sit in front of a screen. Secondly, close your eyes for 20-30 seconds every 20-30 minutes. These simple steps reduce evaporation and promote adequate spread of tears across the eyes. If your eyes still feel tired at the end of the day, remove the lenses during your lunch hour for 30 minutes or so. You can then wear them again for another 8 hours, instead of wearing them for 16 hours at a stretch.

You may temporarily use lubricant eye drops which are over-the-counter medications. They can be safely put in the eye even with the contact lens in place. You can decide the frequency of instillation – they give tremendous comfort, increase your wearing time and reduce your soreness when you remove the lenses. Splashing tap water in the eye after removing the lens is not such a great idea. Putting these sterile artificial tear drops is a better bet!

Q. If I am happy with my lenses, do I need to see an eye doctor at all? Why not buy my replacement lenses directly from the shop?

A. You should see your eye doctor at least once a year, even if you have no problem with your lenses. Ideally, your lenses should be off for at least 48 hours before you visit him. This enables him to recheck your spectacle/contact lens number with greater accuracy. He also looks for early signs of trouble such as growth of blood vessels towards your cornea, dryness, allergy etc. He also examines your retina closely – a procedure which only he is trained to do. All myopes or shortsighted people are at greater risk of developing retinal problems such as retinal holes, tears and even retinal detachments. The risk remains the same, whether you are wearing glasses or contact lenses. As they say, a stitch in time saves nine!

Q. I am over 40 years of age and have used contact lenses throughout my adult life. Can I get bifocal contact lenses?

A. Yes, bifocal lenses are available in India for an increasing range of powers. They take a little while getting used to but are a good option for those above 40 who need reading glasses over their lenses.

Q. Can I wear lenses if I have keratoconus?

A. Keratoconus is a condition of the eye in which the cornea assumes a conical shape. It manifests in your teens and may progress or remain stationary. In the early stages, glasses give adequate vision. However, as the cone becomes steeper, the quality of vision with glasses leaves much to be desired. These can be corrected with the regular use of contact lenses initially. When the regular lenses, too, do not work, various specialty contact lenses are available, such as "Rose-K" lenses, piggyback lenses, scleral lenses etc. However, you need to have a detailed discussion with your eye doctor who will determine which lens is best suited for your eye condition.

Corneal Transplant

Q. What is the 'cornea'?

A. The cornea is the clear tissue that fits like a watch crystal over the iris, the coloured part of the eye. Light passes through the transparent cornea just like it would through a window, to the back of the eye. The light rays get bent, focusing on the inner lining of the back of the eye called the retina. The retina captures the images like the film of a camera.

Q. Why does the cornea get cloudy?

A. The cornea may become cloudy due to different reasons. When it does, light is not able to pass through the eye resulting in poor vision. It is like looking through a piece of frosted glass. Some of the causes are:

- Infection and injury to the eye.
- Nutritional disorders such as Vitamin A deficiency.
- Reaction to drugs, e.g. Stevens-Johnson Syndrome.
- Degenerations and dystrophies of the cornea (inherited conditions which may cause clouding of the cornea in adults).
- Keratoconus (an irregularity of the shape of the cornea, causing its progressive 'coning'). In this condition, the quality of vision gradually deteriorates even if the cornea is clear. Clouding occurs in the later stages.
- Result of a complication during cataract or glaucoma surgery.

Q. Can my vision be restored if the cornea gets clouded?

A. The only way to restore vision is to replace the cornea with donated healthy corneal tissue. This is done by a surgery called corneal transplant or keratoplasty, in which the central disc of the abnormal cornea is removed and replaced by a piece of a normal cornea obtained from a donor eye.

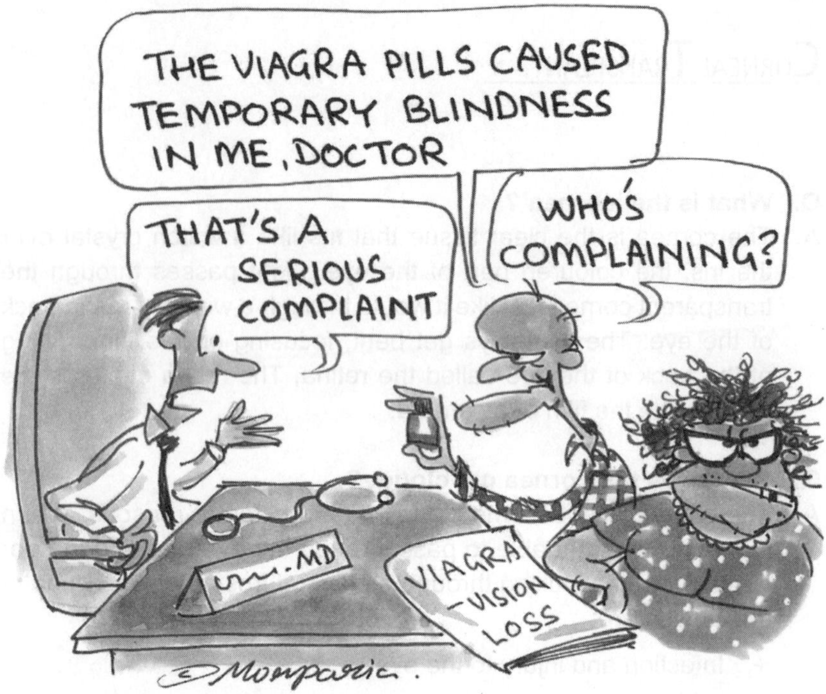
THE VIAGRA PILLS CAUSED TEMPORARY BLINDNESS IN ME, DOCTOR
THAT'S A SERIOUS COMPLAINT
WHO'S COMPLAINING?
VIAGRA -VISION LOSS

Q. How successful is corneal transplant surgery?

A. The cornea is the only part of the eye that can be transplanted. The corneal transplant or corneal graft as it is also called, is not a complicated procedure as the cornea is devoid of blood vessels. Hence it has minimal chances of rejection. I would say it comes second only to hair transplants in terms of success rate!

Even if the transplant is rejected, it can be successfully treated by eye drops in most cases. However, in case a graft does fail or get rejected for some reason and the rejection is not treated in time, all is not lost. If the rest of the eye has no other complications, it is possible to do a regraft after removing the previous opaque graft, thus restoring vision once again.

I have seen several grafts done 30-40 years ago, which remain crystal clear to this day!

Q. When is a corneal transplant rejected?

A. Statistically speaking, rejection occurs most often in the first year after transplant and following any major or minor surgery to the eye thereafter. A patient of corneal graft who undergoes cataract surgery or even removal of his corneal sutures (commonly done a year after the corneal graft surgery) is at increased risk of graft rejection in the month immediately following the surgical procedure.

Q. How will I know that there is early rejection? What should I do?

A. If there is a sudden increase in redness, pain, watering of the operated eye or a decrease in vision in the same eye, you should immediately visit your nearest eye doctor, preferably on the same day. Don't rely on telephonic advice for your symptoms because the same symptoms can occur in graft rejection as well as in graft infection, but the treatment for each is very different.

Q. Under what conditions can a corneal graft fail to restore vision?

A. The following conditions are less suitable for corneal transplants:

- ✦ Grafts done in eyes where the cornea is already vascularised (corneas with blood vessels already growing into them) have a poorer long-term prognosis.
- ✦ Eyes which have a history of previous rejected grafts are more likely to reject again as the body's white blood 'killer' cells mark it as an intruder!
- ✦ Eyes with inadequate tear secretion or with poor quality tears.
- ✦ Any condition that has destroyed the "limbus" i.e. the factory situated at the junction between the black and the white of the eye that constantly replenishes the cells on the surface of the cornea.
- ✦ Chemical burn injuries, drug reactions such as Stevens-Johnson syndrome, which destroy the stem cells of the limbus.
- ✦ Certain congenital conditions such as Aniridia in which there is a very poor quota of stem cells to begin with. (For more information on stem cells, read the chapter on 'Ocular Surface Disorders').

Q. What is 'lamellar' corneal transplant or keratoplasty?

A. Most corneal transplants done in India and the world are 'full thickness' corneal transplants, technically called penetrating keratoplasty. The diseased cornea is removed with all its layers and replaced by a similar or slightly larger-sized donor cornea also of 'full' thickness.

In certain diseases, such as 'Keratoconus' (conical cornea) or in superficial corneal scars, the innermost lining of the cornea called the endothelium is intact and healthy and therefore need not be changed. In such cases, approximately 90% of the thickness is changed, but the innermost layer, the endothelium is left intact. Since it is the donor endothelium which mainly triggers the rejection response by the patient's immune system, the chances of rejection of this 'lamellar' graft are reduced dramatically.

This procedure requires more skill than the usual penetrating keratoplasty and has a 5-10% rate of surgical complications even in the best of hands. DALK (deep anterior lamellar keratoplasty) cannot be used in patients who have an unhealthy endothelium. It therefore requires careful patient selection.

Q. What is "Endothelial Keratoplasty"?

A. Also known as DSEK and DSAEK, endothelial keratoplasty is even more technically demanding than DALK. It requires special instruments and is not routinely done. In this procedure, only the inner lining of the cornea – the endothelium – is transplanted after stripping off the patient's own inner lining. It is performed on patients in whom only the corneal endothelium is dysfunctional, while the rest of the cornea is fine. As sutures are generally not required in such cases, suture-related complications are eliminated and visual recovery is much faster.

Q. What if I have a diseased cornea but cannot undergo or benefit from a cornea transplant?

A. You can be fitted with an artificial cornea or Keratoprosthesis. Please read the chapter devoted to the subject for more information.

Q. What are the expenses involved in corneal transplantation?

A. Expenses vary considerably depending on where you get the surgery done. In India, these surgeries are usually done only in government, municipal or trust hospitals at no charge or a minimal cost. In larger cities, it is done in the private sector as well. Though the eyeball is donated free of cost, most eye banks run extensive tests on the donated tissue as well as test the donor's blood for AIDS, hepatitis and other communicable diseases. They also employ highly-qualified personnel who evaluate the eyeball to decide whether it can be used. All this costs money, which is levied by the eye bank as "processing charges".

In Mumbai for example, it costs around Rs.5000/- per patient. This charge is levied upon patients in the private sector only, who form 30% of all patients receiving donated corneas in Mumbai. The remaining 70% of corneas are distributed practically free of cost to the municipal and free hospitals in the city.

Q. Why does the surgeon charge a fee if the eyeball is procured free from the deceased donor?

A. The professional fee charged by an eye surgeon is usually similar to what he would charge for a cataract surgery. Though the eyeball comes free, the surgeon uses good surgical microscopes, disposable trephines, other costly tools and above all, his expertise to perform a successful corneal grafting surgery. Moreover, most eye surgeons use the income from patients who can pay to subsidise the surgery for those who cannot afford it.

Q. Can every blind person regain sight by a corneal transplant?

A. No. Corneal transplant surgery can only benefit those who are blind due to the cornea becoming opaque. The rest of the eye tissues cannot be transplanted. As of today, retinal transplants are being tried on an experimental basis but it will be many years if at all, before this procedure can be performed successfully to restore vision to those with diseased retinas.

Q. Can a person who has received a corneal transplant himself donate his cornea after death?

A. Yes. If the cornea is clear, it can be re-used to give sight to another corneally blind person. It would be a truly noble gesture!

Diabetes, Hypertension and The Eye

Q. Why should I care about diabetes?

A. Did you know that India has perhaps the world's second-largest population of diabetics? The number of new diabetics is growing by leaps and bounds. This is due in large measure to our aping the couch potato culture of the west and their junk food habits. Similarly, hypertension or high blood pressure, which was earlier restricted to Type A personalities (perfectionists, high achievers etc.) is increasingly affecting the urban poor as well as the rural population.

Q. How can diabetes affect my eyes?

A. If you have been a diabetic for 20 years, you have greater than 50% chance of developing eye problems, even though you have had it in superb control for all those years! Your risk however increases even further if you have been a 'naughty' diabetic who has paid scant regard to your doctor's advice on diet, medication and exercise.

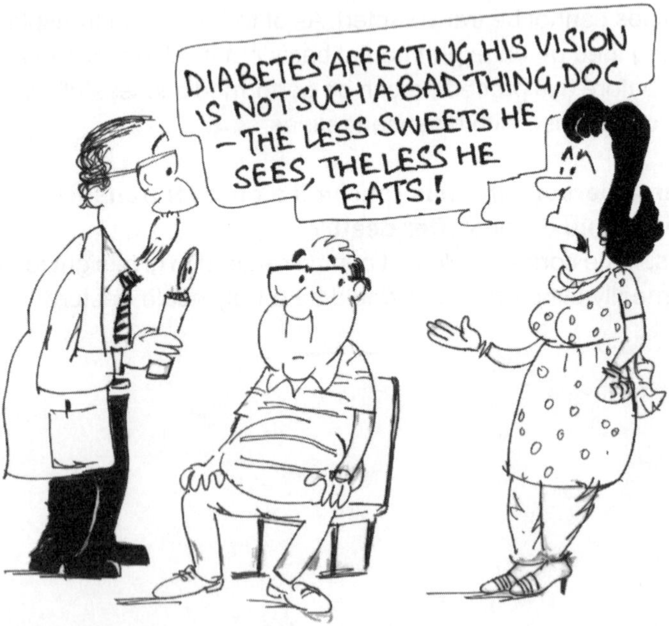
DIABETES AFFECTING HIS VISION IS NOT SUCH A BAD THING, DOC – THE LESS SWEETS HE SEES, THE LESS HE EATS!

Diabetes commonly causes retinal problems, glaucoma, cataract and increases the risk of eye infections. Other, less common problems are paralysis of one or more eye muscles, dry eye and affections of the optic nerve (the nerve of sight).

Q. How often should I get my eyes examined if I am diabetic or hypertensive?

A. As soon as you become aware of your diabetes or hypertension, you should have a complete eye examination. If your condition has not affected the eye, your eye doctor may recommend annual visits. But if you are detected with any diabetic or hypertensive eye disease you will have to visit him more often.

Q. What will my eye doctor check for once he knows I am diabetic?

A. Since diabetics are more prone to various eye afflictions, your doctor will not only look at the retina, but will also check the pressure of the eye, rule out glaucoma, examine the eye on a slit lamp biomicroscope to rule out early cataracts and test you for dry eye. The adage 'a stitch in time saves nine' was probably written for a diabetic!

Q. Can I not simply wait till I develop some eye symptoms before I visit an eye specialist?

A. That may be being penny-wise and pound-foolish. Many a problem can be detected and treated even before symptoms develop. Treating it later may be more expensive and worse, less effective!

Q. Can an eye doctor detect diabetes or hypertension simply by checking my eyes?

A. Yes. The blood vessels of the retina mirror the changes taking place in the rest of the body. These are the only blood vessels in the whole body that can be viewed by a simple non-invasive technique (ophthalmoscopy). That is why an eye doctor can tell if you are a diabetic or hypertensive simply by examining your retina! If your retinal blood vessels show progressive changes of diabetes or hypertension, he can warn you to discuss stricter control with your treating physician.

Q. What kind of retinal problems (retinopathy) do diabetics face?

A. The tiny retinal blood vessels in diabetics are more prone to leakages:

- ✦ Retinal haemorrhage – leakage of blood into the retina
- ✦ Vitreous haemorrhage – leakage of blood into the jelly of the eye in front of the retina.
- ✦ Macular oedema – leakage of fluid containing proteins into the retina, collecting in the centre i.e. the macular area.
- ✦ Leakage of fatty material, cholesterol etc into the retina, either in the centre or in the periphery.

Any form of leakage in the macular area will result in distorted vision or a drop in vision. This may be sudden, such as when bleeding occurs, or gradual, when fluid oozes slowly into the macular area.

Q. What should I do when my vision begins to fail?

A. As a diabetic, you should learn how to examine your vision at home at regular intervals, covering one eye at a time. You should do it with correct glasses, for both distance and near. Visit your eye doctor, the moment you detect a fall in vision.

Chances are you may not notice anything amiss until much later if the leakages are not in the centre of the retina. Therefore it is essential that you visit the eye doctor regularly. The eye doctor will dilate your pupils and carefully examine the macula and periphery of the retina using an instrument called an ophthalmoscope. If he does detect leakages, he may conduct a fluorescein angiography test to detect the site of the leakages and then use a laser to treat them.

Q. Will use of the laser cure my diabetic retinopathy?

A. The aim of laser treatment is to preserve whatever vision there is left, not improve it. As the diabetes progresses, especially if it is poorly controlled, fresh haemorrhages and leakages can occur. This may necessitate repeated laser treatments. Unfortunately, our retinal cells do not grow. Hence, damaged cells will result in permanent loss of vision in the affected area.

Q. I have heard of some new drugs which can be injected into the eye to improve my vision. Are they useful?

A. In certain cases, diabetes affects the central area of the retina, called the macula, increasing its thickness and resulting in poor central vision. These can now be treated with intra-vitreal injections of certain new drugs into the jelly in front of the retina. These are usually given as a course of 3 injections at intervals of 4-6 weeks. The injections have shown good results in select cases, even improving patients' vision. These new drugs are expensive but as more and more doctors use them, they are becoming cheaper.

Q. What will happen if I ignore the doctor's advice or delay the treatment?

A. This is a very common tactic employed by patients – I call it the 'ostrich' approach. Stick your head in the sand and pretend the problem is not there, or will not affect you, or will somehow become better with time! Unfortunately, eye problems only get aggravated if not tackled in time. In diabetic retinopathy (affection of the retina), haemorrhages and/or cholesterol deposits on the surface of the retina can gradually lead to the formation of new, fragile tiny blood vessels in the retina, which repeatedly burst, giving rise to fresh haemorrhages. If the vessels burst into the jelly in front of the retina, giving rise to a vitreous haemorrhage, you will experience a tremendous drop in vision. Worse still, formation of natural scar tissue may cause a pull or traction on the retina causing a traction retinal detachment. Proliferation of these new vessels on the retina or into the vitreous is known as proliferative vitreo-retinopathy. This condition requires complicated vitreoretinal surgery, which may not give good results. In the worst case scenario, you could go blind!

In most cases, timely intervention during the early stages can arrest or at least markedly delay the progression of the disease to the next stage. All it takes is for you to visit your eye doctor at regular intervals as advised, so that the retina can be examined properly.

Q. What precautions should I should take with my diabetic or hypertensive medications in case I am advised eye surgery?

A. We usually recommend the discontinuation of oral anti-diabetic medication on the morning of surgery. You may resume the medication along with your next major meal. In case you are on insulin, you should follow the advice of your diabetes specialist. You should inform your physician about the time of surgery, so that he can alter your insulin schedule accordingly. Most eye surgery is done under local anaesthesia, hence you need not starve yourself before the surgery.

If you are hypertensive, it is very important that you continue your medications as per schedule and not miss a single dose, especially on the morning of the surgery. You should inform your eye doctor about your condition and the medications you are on. He may avoid the use of adrenaline and similar compounds during surgery as they may cause a rise in blood pressure.

Ocular Surface Disorders

Q. What is the ocular surface?

A. The ocular surface is basically the outer surface of the eye. It consists of:

- The conjunctiva, which is the transparent, thin layer that lines the inner surface of the two eyelids and covers the white of the eye.
- The white portion of the eye called the sclera.
- The cornea, which is the transparent cover over the brown/ black of the eye. Composed of several layers, its topmost layer called the corneal epithelium is part of this ocular surface.
- The limbus, which is the junction of the sclera and the cornea. This area contains stem cells which are precursor cells that differentiate throughout life to create new surface cells of the conjunctiva on the one side and the epithelial cells of the cornea on the other. When the limbus gets damaged, conjunctival and corneal cells do not get replaced properly, resulting in surface disorders.
- The tear film produced by the lachrymal glands. Part of the tear film is also produced by glands in the eyelids (oily part of tears) and a part by cells in the conjunctiva (sticky, mucus part of the tears).

Q. Why are tears important?

A. The tear film lubricates the ocular surface and protects it by washing away harmful substances. We do not realize it, but it is produced continuously. The tears we shed when we see the hero or heroine being hammered in a Bollywood movie are "emotional tears". These are different in composition from your regular lubricating tears and are of no use whatsoever in moistening the ocular surface. Hence you may shed copious tears at the drop of a hat and yet be diagnosed with a 'dry eye'!

Q. How does one develop dry eye?

A. Tear production decreases with age. A 60-year-old produces 60%

less tears than an average 18-year-old. Some of the common causes of dry eye are:

- ✦ Menopause and pregnancy.
- ✦ Staring continuously at the computer screen without blinking. When you do not blink adequately, tears do not spread evenly across the ocular surface and more tears evaporate from the surface of the eye, thus causing dry eye.
- ✦ Prolonged use of contact lenses.
- ✦ Allopathic drugs such as antihistamines (taken for common colds), antacids, anti-hypertensives, anti-depressants, drugs used for Parkinson's disease and various other medications.
- ✦ Certain environments such as windy, dusty, dry climates and atmospheric pollution. Also, overuse of heaters (less likely in most parts of India) and air-conditioners (most likely in most parts of India) causes the room air to become dry, promoting evaporation of our tears.

Q. How is dry eye treated?

A. Generally, tear substitutes in the form of drops or ointments or both, depending on the severity, are given to treat dry eye. In some cases, the eye surgeon may advise blockage of the tear drainage ducts so as to preserve the patient's own tears in the eye for a longer time as well as to lessen the need for using artificial tears.

Q. My cousin was advised "occlusion of his puncti" to relieve his dry eye. What does it mean?

A. In mild to moderate dry eye cases, we try to conserve the patient's own tears as much as possible. There are tiny openings in the medial edge of our upper and lower eyelids (near the nose) called 'puncti'. Our tears normally drain out from these puncti into tiny canals called canaliculi into the lachrymal sac and from there into the nose through another canal called the nasolachrymal duct.

By blocking the 'puncti' with plugs, much like the blocking of the washbasin drain with a rubber bung, we reduce the amount of the patient's own tears going 'down the drain'! Therefore more of the patient's own tears are available to lubricate his eye, reducing his dependence on lubricant drops and ointments.

There are mainly two types of 'plugs' available in the market:

- 'Punctum' plugs, which are inserted into the tiny openings in the upper and lower lids through which our tears drain and remain visible on the surface of the lid and
- Canalicular plugs, which are inserted through the puncti into the drainage pathway and are therefore not visible to the naked eye once inserted.

Both these types are inserted in an easy, no-injection technique using only eyedrop anaesthesia.

Q. Why can't we use plugs in every case of 'dry eye'?

A. In severe forms of dry eye, the quality of the patient's own tears is not good. In such cases, allowing the patient's own tears (however small in quantity they may be) to remain in the eye for longer periods may do more harm than good.

Q. Can something be done for a virtually blind patient with severe dry eye and opaque cornea?

A. Yes, a device called keratoprosthesis or artificial cornea can be inserted even in bone-dry eyes with opaque and vascularised corneas and the patient can regain his vision. This is a major surgery, often done in two stages and performed by only a handful of eye surgeons in the country. It should be undertaken as a last resort only after careful consideration of each individual case. (See chapter on keratoprosthesis)

Q. What is an amniotic membrane transplant?

A. Sometimes the ocular surface gets damaged by complications like non-healing corneal ulcers (breaks in the superficial layer of the cornea due to infection), large perforations of the cornea, surface irregularities of the ocular surface such as after removing surface tumours, or ocular traumas due to acids, alkalis or other toxic substances. In such cases, the ocular surface needs a new cover, which can be provided by a biological tissue like amnion.

The amniotic membrane is the inner lining of the protective cover of the foetus in a mother's womb. After a Caesarian section in a volunteer, the amniotic membrane is carefully stripped off from the placenta and preserved in a special medium for 6 months. The donor is tested for various blood-borne diseases including AIDS. These tests are repeated after 6 months and if negative, the amniotic tissue is used for covering the ocular surface.

This surgery was very popular in the fifties and sixties and has found favour again in the last decade.

Q. How long does the amniotic membrane (AM) stay in place?

A. This depends on how inflamed or 'angry' the eye is. The more inflamed the eye, the faster the amniotic membrane is absorbed – sometimes even as fast as one week. If there is not much inflammation, the AM may continue to provide protection for 4-6 weeks.

Q. What is corneal glue? When is it used?

A. In case there is a tiny hole in the cornea following injury or melting of the cornea due to chemical burns or infection, a glue similar to Fevicol or Araldite is used to seal the opening. This is a medical grade polymer; a drop or two is all that is required. It is a quick-drying glue but also an extreme irritant. Hence, after it has dried on the cornea, a bandage contact lens is applied to keep the glue in place and to prevent the severe irritation that the patient would feel if the glue came in contact with his eyelids.

Q. Is it true that the eye produces stem cells?

A. Yes. Just like our skin, the cornea and the conjunctiva continuously shed and replace their surface layer of cells with new cells. Until recently, we were not sure where these new cells came from. It has now been proved that the limbus i.e. the junction of the cornea and the sclera (the white of the eye) is home to stem cells. These limbal stem cells form the new epithelial cells of the cornea and conjunctiva.

The beauty of it all is that each stem cell divides into two daughter stem cells. While one remains the same, the other goes on to differentiate into the corneal and conjunctival cells, which ultimately die and are cast off. This process goes on throughout the individual's life, thus providing a continual supply of new cells for the cornea without a significant drop in the total stem cell population.

Q. What happens if the stem cells of the eye are damaged?

A. The stem cells of the eye can get damaged by certain diseases and chemical (acid burn) injuries. Then the regular cast-off cells from the surface of the cornea are no longer replaced by stem cells, resulting in persistent defects in the epithelial layer of the cornea.

With time, this results in loss of transparency of the cornea and drop in vision. Until recently, these eyes were given up for lost. Even a corneal transplant was doomed to failure in such cases, as the superficial cells of the new donated cornea would soon be cast off but not replaced due to the stem cell deficiency of the patient.

Q. Can stem cells help to restore vision?

A. Yes. If one eye is damaged, stem cells can be harvested from the limbus of the second eye. This tissue containing the stem cells can be then transplanted into the diseased eye. The stem cells soon start dividing and subdividing and fill up the defects in the recipient cornea. Eyes with very poor vision can have their vision restored by this simple procedure.

Q. What if both eyes are similarly damaged or diseased?

A. All is not lost. Even if a tiny area of normal stem cells is available in either eye, a part of it can be removed and cultured in the laboratory. In a couple of weeks, this tiny bit of tissue can be made to grow to several times its original size i.e. from a few stem cells to several hundreds of stem cells. This newly-grown tissue can then be transplanted into one or both eyes. Over a period of time, one or both corneas can regain sufficient number of cells to improve vision.

Q. What if both eyes are so damaged that stem cells cannot be harvested from either?

A. In such cases, stem cells can be harvested from a sibling or parent and transplanted into any one eye of the patient. In case they are unwilling, not available or not found suitable, then stem cells can be harvested from an unrelated cadaveric donated eye i.e. from a dead donor. In both these cases however, there is always the fear of rejection, hence such patients are given immunosuppressive drugs for a prolonged period of time.

Eye Donation

Q. Who can be an eye donor?

A. Anyone can be an eye donor, irrespective of age, sex, religion, caste, creed or blood group.

Q. Do all religions allow eye donation?

A. Yes, all religions support eye donation.

Q. Is the whole eye used for transplant?

A. No, only the thin transparent layer in front of the iris called the cornea is used to replace the diseased or opaque cornea in the eye of the patient (recipient).

Q. Do cataracts or the use of spectacles render the cornea unfit for donation?

A. No, both these conditions relate to the lens of the eye and not the cornea. In fact, people who have been successfully operated for cataracts or glaucoma or even retinal detachments can also donate their eyes after death. In fact there have been instances of those who have received a corneal transplant themselves donating their corneas after death! All that is required is that the donor has a clear, transparent, healthy cornea at the time of death.

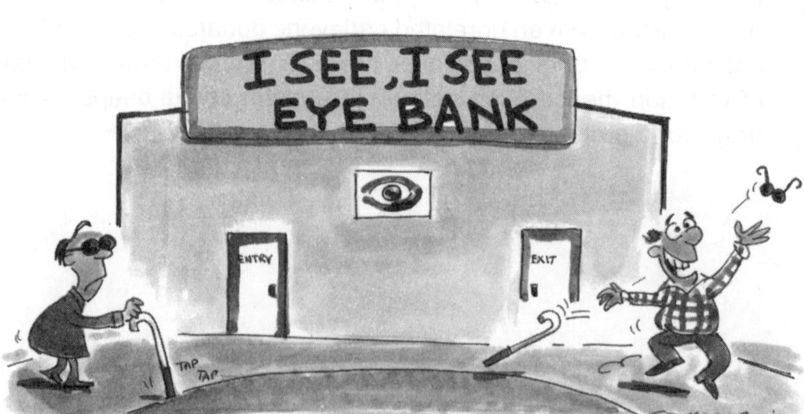

Q. Does eye donation disfigure the donor's face?

A. No, the removal of the eyes neither disfigures the face nor interferes with the customary funeral arrangements.

Q. Does the human body reject the transplanted donor's cornea?

A. The human cornea does not have any blood supply; hence the risk of rejection is very low. Rejection, if it does occur, can be suppressed by timely medication.

Q. How successful are corneal transplants?

A. In general, the chances of success are greater than 80%. In deep anterior lamellar transplants, where the inner lining of the cornea called the endothelium is not transplanted, the success rate is as high as 95%!

Q. What conditions render the cornea unfit for donation?

A. Corneas of people suffering from AIDS, rabies, syphillis, tetanus, septicaemia and certain viral diseases cannot be transplanted. People with diabetes, hypertension or cancer can donate their eyes. However, if the donor had blood-borne cancer then the cornea of such a patient cannot be used.

Q. Is there any use for corneas which are deemed unfit for transplant?

A. Corneas, which for some reason cannot be used for corneal transplants, are invaluable for research and training programmes.

Q. What is done with the eyes that are removed from a donor?

A. After the eyes are removed, they are evaluated, processed, screened by an eye bank and then supplied to the eye surgeon for transplant.

Q. Do corneal transplants guarantee sight to all blind people?

A. No, transplants only help when the loss of sight is solely due to corneal defects and the rest of the eye mechanism is intact.

Q. How quickly should the eyes be removed after death?

A. As soon as possible, but eyes can be removed up to 6 hours after death. However, in places where the climate is hot such as in most parts of India, a shorter duration, preferably 2 to 4 hours after death is advisable.

Q. Is it necessary to take the donor to the hospital after death?

A. No, eye banks have personnel who will come to the donor's home or place of death and remove the eyes.

Q. What is an eye bank?

A. An eye bank is the link between the donor and recipient/eye surgeon. It is an organization authorised by the government to collect and distribute human eyes to those who require corneal transplants.

Q. What is to be done when a relative expires?

A. The following steps ease the procedure of removing a donor's eyes after death.

- Keep the death certificate or its copy to show to the eye bank team. They do not need a photocopy of the same in the middle of the night. The team only needs to look at the certificate to determine:
  - a) The patient is really dead and
  - b) The cause of death, to determine if the eyeball can be useful.
- Contact your nearest eye bank – the eye bank contact number in most Indian cities is 1919. Otherwise, check the local telephone directory – most eye banks are listed in the emergency numbers list. The eye bank team will arrive in the next 30-60 minutes, provided you have given them an accurate address with landmarks. The procedure takes only around 30-40 minutes.
- Close the eye lids, while waiting for the eye bank team and put off any overhead fan to prevent drying of the cornea. However, you may switch on an air-conditioner, if possible.
- If possible, cover the closed lids with moist cotton wool.
- Raise the donor's head by 6 inches, by placing two pillows under it.

Q. Is blood also collected during the procedure?

A. Yes, according to WHO guidelines, the team will also collect some blood from the donor, to test for HIV, hepatitis etc. They will withdraw this from a large blood vessel or from the heart using a needle puncture.

Q. Is there any cumbersome paperwork or does one need to complete time-consuming formalities?

A. None whatsoever. The eye bank team will come with a form, which they will fill themselves. They will only need the signatures of two close relatives giving consent. It does not matter whether the donor had pledged his eyes for donation during his lifetime or not.

Q. Finally, is there any money to be paid?

A. No, there is no monetary transaction. Most eye banks recover their running costs by charging the recipients a small processing fee.

Q. If eye donation is so easy, and encouraged by every religion, why aren't there more donors?

A. Good question. You tell me! You go around spreading the message of the nobility of eye donation (better still ask friends to pay and purchase this book and read this chapter themselves!) and how easy and hassle-free it is and maybe by the time I write the next edition, this question will need deletion!

GLAUCOMA

Q. What is glaucoma?

A. Simply put, it is a disease in which the pressure inside the eye is more than the eye can tolerate. If the pressure continues to remain high, the optic nerve of the eye, which is sensitive to pressure, starts deteriorating gradually.

Q. Who is at greater risk of developing glaucoma?

A. No one is immune from glaucoma. However, those with a family history of glaucoma, ocular trauma, diabetes, high blood pressure, small eyes with narrow angles, minus number glasses and those who are elderly are more prone to developing glaucoma. This disease usually develops after the age of 40, hence you must undergo an annual eye check-up after reaching 40. But if you fall into any of the risk categories mentioned above, you should start the annual check-up at an earlier age.

Q. What are the symptoms of glaucoma?

A. Unfortunately, there are no symptoms in a majority of cases. The field of vision starts constricting gradually from the periphery towards the centre until only a tubular field is left. The patient starts bumping into objects or stumbling frequently over uneven pavements. Most elderly patients usually ascribe their diminishing vision to cataract and delay visiting their eye doctors. What they don't realize is that though the central vision is fine, the peripheral field is being irreversibly lost to glaucoma. Little wonder then, that glaucoma is called the 'silent thief of vision'.

Patients who suffer from 'narrow angle glaucoma' may experience early symptoms like frequent change of glasses, headaches, occasional redness of the eyes etc. These patients may also suffer a 'glaucoma attack' with severe pain, redness and watering of the eye accompanied by nausea or even vomiting.

Q. Can my optician not diagnose glaucoma?

A. No. Though your optician is excellent for checking your numbers, he is not trained to diagnose eye diseases. An ophthalmologist alone is equipped to diagnose glaucoma. You need to visit your eye doctor at least once at age of 40 and then ideally annually thereafter.

Q. How does an eye surgeon detect glaucoma?

A. Your eye surgeon will take your eye pressure, either in the lying down position (Schiotz tonometry) or in the sitting up position (applanation tonometry, non-contact or minimal contact tonometry). Though an isolated high reading need not indicate glaucoma, your ophthalmologist will look closely at your optic nerve (the only nerve of the brain visible to a doctor) through an instrument called an ophthalmoscope. If the nerve looks like it is getting compromised or pressed upon, he may record his findings in drawings or photographs. He may also study the loss of peripheral vision by doing a computerized visual field examination.

Glaucoma is known to affect the ability to distinguish between objects of low contrast. Hence contrast sensitivity tests are conducted to better diagnose early glaucoma. Open-angled glaucoma is distinguished from narrow-angled glaucoma by studying the angle of the eye (the area from which the fluid of the eye exits) with a contact lens known as a gonioscope. Other high tech tests for difficult-to-diagnose cases include Optical Coherence Tomography (OCT) and Nerve Fibre Analyzers.

Q. Is there a medical cure for glaucoma?

A. Like diabetes, glaucoma can be kept under control in most cases with the help of drugs. Initially, you may need to take oral tablets for a short time and then you only need to put an eye drop once or twice a day. Your eye surgeon will determine the 'target pressure' that is safe for your eye and will try to keep your eye pressure at or below that 'target pressure' to prevent damage to the optic nerve. He will monitor this by checking your pressure, examining the optic nerve and checking your visual fields at regular intervals. Depending on these parameters, he may change or add new eye drops from time to time. Alternatively, he may resort to surgery if he is not happy with the response of your eye to medical therapy.

Q. How safe is surgery?

A. Glaucoma surgery is fairly safe and free of complications. The surgeon raises a flap of the sclera (white of the eye) and makes a new drainage pathway for the fluid of the eye to escape. This flap is then closed with stitches, which may or may not require removal. This surgery is known as trabeculectomy.

Q. Will I develop a cataract after glaucoma surgery?

A. Trabeculectomy does hasten the onset of cataract in some patients. You must remember though, that glaucoma patients are elderly and usually develop a cataract in their lenses even before surgery. Modern cataract surgery is safe and effective in eyes previously operated upon for glaucoma. If you have a significant amount of cataract and glaucoma, your eye surgeon may do a combined glaucoma and cataract surgery with an intra-ocular lens implant, all in one sitting.

Q. I want to avoid surgery. What about laser treatment?

A. Lasers are indeed used to treat glaucoma. If the angle of your eye is narrow, you may develop an acute attack of glaucoma. To prevent such an attack, a laser can be used to make a small hole in the brown of your eye (peripheral iridectomy). This however, does not cure your glaucoma.

In open-angled glaucoma, a laser is used to widen the openings in the angle for fluid to drain out, thus reducing the pressure. However, most eye surgeons increasingly view this as a temporary measure, rarely being effective beyond five years at best.

Q. Are there newer surgical procedures which are safer than trabeculectomy?

A. Since the last decade or so, a few new procedures have been developed which are "non-penetrating", i.e. the anterior chamber of the eye is not penetrated. They are supposed to avoid the danger of causing too low a pressure after surgery. However, these procedures have a marginally lower percentage of success in the long run.

Q. What are glaucoma valves?

A. Glaucoma valves are artificial, usually plastic (PMMA) devices which have a tube placed in the eye's anterior chamber with a valve at the end of the tube. This allows fluid to drain from the eye when the pressure is high and blocks the drainage when pressure is normal or low, thus maintaining adequate eye pressure. The use of glaucoma valves has shown great promise in patients in whom trabeculectomy has not worked or will not work. Earlier they were used only in failed glaucoma operated cases, but now they are also used as a primary procedure in select cases.

Q. Does surgery guarantee a cure for glaucoma and lifetime freedom from glaucoma medication?

A. I wish it were true. In 80-90% of cases, the visual fields may stop deteriorating and the pressure may remain below target forever. However there is a 10-20% possibility of the pressure remaining uncontrolled or visual fields continuing to worsen even after uneventful surgery. This may happen immediately after surgery or even several years after seeming 'cure'. Therefore, even after successful surgery you should continue to see your eye surgeon at regular intervals as called, to confirm, "All is still well"! More importantly, we must realize that at best, surgery can only prevent further loss of vision – it cannot restore vision already lost, unlike cataract surgery. In other words, delaying glaucoma treatment, medical or surgical, is like going down a one-way street – there is no coming back!

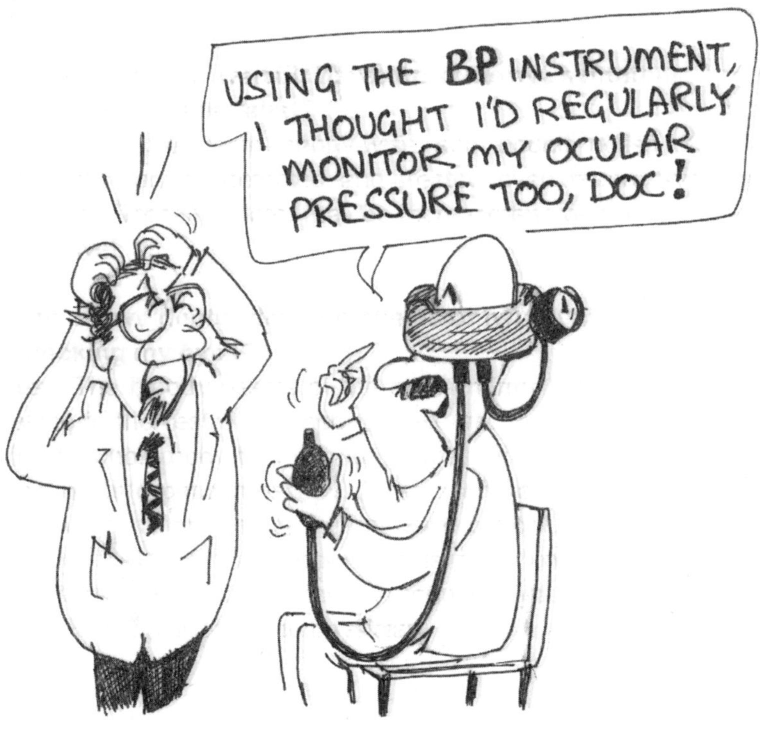
USING THE BP INSTRUMENT, I THOUGHT I'D REGULARLY MONITOR MY OCULAR PRESSURE TOO, DOC!

Q. What is the role of diet and exercise in glaucoma?

A. Several recent studies cite excess intake of caffeine as a risk factor for glaucoma. On the other hand, regular exercise such as walking, swimming, jogging is known to be beneficial in controlling glaucoma.

Q. Can a person who has undergone glaucoma surgery donate his eyes after death?

A. Most certainly, provided the cornea is clear.

LASER REMOVAL OF EYE NUMBERS

Q. What kind of laser is used for removing eye numbers?

A. It is known as the Excimer laser. The most common method used is LASIK. In this method, a partial thickness hinged flap (approximately 90-160 microns thick) is raised (somewhat like opening a Pepsi/Coke/Thums Up can – I have no shares in any of the 3 companies!) Laser is then applied to the bed of the cornea, removing minute amounts of tissue at each laser shot. The number of shots varies with the patient's spectacle number and is pre-determined by the machine's built-in computer after the eye surgeon has fed correct data into it. After the procedure, the surgeon gently puts back the hinged flap, which falls perfectly into place. Minutes later, the flap is well-fused with the rest of the cornea and will not dislodge even under moderate stress. The surgeon then goes on to perform LASIK on the second eye.

Q. My nine-year-old daughter's number keeps increasing every few months. Can she undergo the LASIK procedure?

A. No. LASIK is only done for those whose spectacle number is stable i.e. it has not increased in the last one year. As per US FDA guidelines, the patient should be at least 18 years old because the number can keep increasing till 18 in a majority of short-sighted individuals. However, it may stabilize in your daughter's case at 24; in that case, we will do LASIK for her when she is 24 years old!

Q. Is LASIK only for those with minus numbers?

A. No, it can be done for those with all types of numbers - myopes (minus numbers), hypermetropes (plus numbers) and astigmatics (those with cylindrical numbers, plus or minus) – provided they have a stable number and are at least 18 years old.

Exceptions are sometimes made for children having a high stable number in only one eye. That eye becomes amblyopic (lazy) if not used. If the child cannot tolerate spectacles or contact lenses in one eye, LASIK is offered by some surgeons as an option.

Q. Is LASIK safe?

A. Someone in the West stated that LASIK is safer than driving or walking on the roads! More than 95% of patients will have virtually no complications after LASIK, when done after careful patient selection and using standard techniques. Of the remaining 5%, the complications in most cases are minor, reversible or curable with treatment and not sight-threatening. Rarely do patients develop sight-threatening complications.

Q. What are the common complications of LASIK procedures?

A. Complications affect less than 5% of LASIK patients. The most common complications are under-correction and over-correction. This is because all LASIK machines use complex computer calculations, based on the data of thousands of patients, to determine how much of the corneal stroma should be shaved to achieve the desired result. However your eye may not heal the same way as an average eye, leading to an under-correction or over-correction. Luckily, in almost all cases, it occurs within the first year, after which the vision remains stable.

Usually the amount of residual refractive error is 0.5 or less, which is quite compatible with normal vision and nothing further needs to be done. In case you are left with +/- 1.0 or greater, it can be corrected by repeating the laser treatment at no extra cost if done within the first year of treatment. LASIK specialists call this touch-up treatment an 'enhancement procedure'!

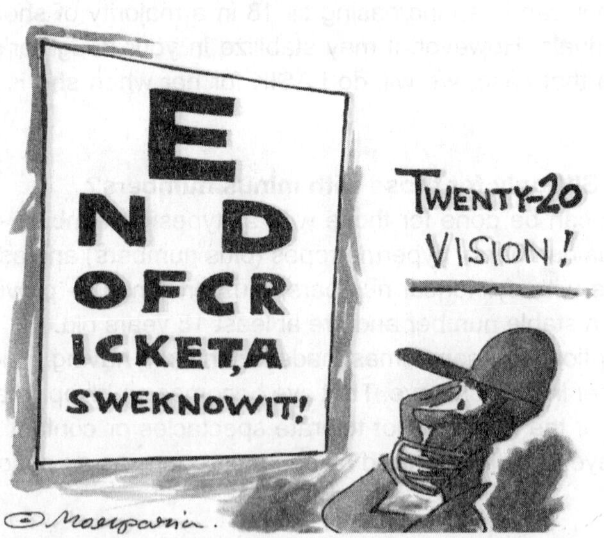

Q. My mother developed dry eye after a LASIK procedure. Is that normal? Will she face other complications?

A. Besides under- and over-correction, there are other not-so-common complications. A patient can develop dry eye i.e. a lessening of his normal tear production, needing the use of lubricant eye drops for up to a couple of months. This problem usually resolves over time.

In Western countries, patients generally have large pupils, which dilate more than ours in semi-darkness. They may face glare, difficulty in night-driving and haloes around light. These problems are rarely seen in Indians.

Since the lifting of the flap is a surgical procedure, there is the theoretical chance of infection if adequate sterilization precautions are not taken. Most LASIK surgeons prescribe topical antibiotics for a week or two after the procedure as a preventive measure. In rare instances, patients may face flap-related complications such as a 'free' cap i.e. the flap may become unhinged. However, modern keratomes have built in safety features to prevent this complication.

Q. What are 'higher-order aberrations' of the eye? Can they be treated by LASIK?

A. Besides spherical and cylindrical numbers, our eyes also have what are technically referred to as 'higher-order aberrations'. The cornea and the lens of the eye bend the incoming light rays so that they focus on the part of the retina that is sensitive to light. This usually induces mild distortions of the light, which were undetectable before aberrometers were invented. These distortions can be corrected by the modern 'wave-front' guided LASIK machines, giving an enhanced quality of vision. As this procedure entails zapping off more tissue than standard LASIK, it is not suitable for all patients.

Ask your LASIK surgeon if you can undergo the procedure. He will perform an aberrometry test to check if you do have significant higher-order aberrations and whether your residual corneal bed at the end of the procedure will be thick enough to do the procedure.

Q. I have heard of a new procedure called 'LASEK'. What is it?

A. LASEK is a procedure for those whose corneas are too thin to remove the full spectacle number. The surgeon reduces the corneal flap to only around 50 microns in thickness instead of the standard 160 microns. This means that he has another 110 microns of cornea available for zapping. However, creating such a thin flap (only the epithelium is peeled off) poses a greater risk of flap-related complications.

Q. What is the Femto-second Laser?

A. This is the latest form of laser, which uses a laser beam to cut the LASIK flap. Others use mechanical 'keratomes' to make the hinged flap. The long-term results of this procedure are not known as it is still a fairly new procedure. So far, the final result with the standard laser and the Femto-second is the same. However, the cost of this machine is very high and the cost of treatment higher.

Q. How soon can I resume my normal activities after LASIK?

A. You will experience mild soreness, watering and discomfort on the first day. You can resume office after 24-48 hours. There is no restriction on any visual activity such as TV, computers or reading following the procedure. Most surgeons will prescribe antibiotics and lubricant drops for a couple of weeks post-surgery along with some mild steroid or non-steroidal anti-inflammatory drops. You should go for your first post-operative check-up within 24 hours after the procedure and then maybe after a week. After this, the surgeon will decide the frequency of post-operative visits.

Q. If my cornea is too thin or my number too high for LASIK, can I still be free of spectacles?

A. Yes. Today, 2-3 designs of intra-ocular lenses are available that can be placed into the eye without removing the patient's own lens. These are known as Phakic IOL and are fairly safe. The lenses need to be specially ordered for your number. However, not all patients are good candidates for the procedure. You should carefully discuss the pros and cons with your surgeon. It is slightly more expensive than LASIK.

Q. I am 55 years old and require glasses only for reading. Can I get rid of my glasses?

A. Yes. These are some of your options:

- If you are prepared to have one eye corrected for near and the other for distance, you can opt to have LASIK in one eye for near correction.

- 'Conductive keratoplasty' uses radio-frequency waves at eight spots in the periphery of the cornea to correct the near spectacle number in one eye.
- A few LASIK surgeons do carry out presbyopic correction by LASIK for both eyes, but it is not yet a standard procedure.
- You can also opt to have 'refractive lens exchange' done on both eyes. In this procedure, your natural lens is surgically removed even before it can turn cataractous and replaced by an artificial multi-focal lens in both eyes, thereby making you independent of glasses both for distance and near. However, this is a surgical procedure, with the theoretical possibility of complications such as haemorrhage, infection and loss of sight.

Q. Can a person who has undergone a LASIK procedure donate his eyes after death?

A. Yes he can. The author is not aware of any such donation actually having been made, however.

Keratoconus

Q. What is Keratoconus (Kconus)?

A. In Keratoconus a cross-section of the cornea assumes a conical shape, compared to the near-spherical shape of the normal cornea. The cornea, incidentally, is the clear transparent structure which sits like a dome over the coloured portion of the eye, much like the glass in front of a wristwatch.

Q. Is Kconus present from birth?

A. No, it usually manifests during the late teens or in the twenties, though it is thought to be due to genetic causes.

Q. How is it suspected by a patient, in the early stages?

A. If the patient is unhappy with the quality of vision with his spectacles, but feels he sees better with a hard contact lens, he needs to be tested for Keratoconus.

Q. What are the tests for Kconus?

A. Until recently, clinical suspicion by the ophthalmologist was the most important. After all, the eye does not see what the mind does not know! He then did a Retinoscopy, or reflected a beam of light into the patient's eye from a distance of one metre. In Kconus, he often found a characteristic "scissors" image being reflected back. He then examined the cornea using highly-magnified slit lamp bio-microscopy, where early change of shape could be picked up.

However, in modern times, there are machines called corneal topographers which document precisely the contour of the cornea, much like terrain mapping in geography. They even issue a warning, telling the eye surgeon that the patient being tested is a "Kconus suspect". In late cases, the cornea thins near the steepest part of the cone. We now have instruments called pachymeters, which measure the thickness of the cornea at various zones of the cornea. An area of unusual thinning would arouse suspicion of Keratoconus.

Q. Are all Kconus cases progressive?

A. Good question. No, only around a quarter (25% for those who are mathematically challenged!) of cases will progress. The progress is usually very slow, over years. In those who also suffer from allergic conjunctivitis (a common association) or frequent "eye rubbers" the rate of progression may be faster.

Q. What is the worst case scenario? Can my cornea "burst'?

A. In a small percentage of progressive cases, the inner layers of the cornea can give way. It is a condition called 'hydrops'. The cornea becomes steamy and opaque as it accumulates water. This condition is usually self-limiting – the imbibed water disappears and the vision can even improve over time.

Q. I have been diagnosed as Kconus and I am unhappy with my spectacles. What next?

A. The answer, in two words is 'contact lenses'. There are several options in contact lens wear for Kconus. Let your doctor decide which is best for you, after trials. You may wear 'hard' contact lenses, which are the smallest contact lenses, sitting only on the cornea. The other lenses are the RGP (rigid-gas permeable) or 'semi-soft' contact lenses, which allow oxygen to enter the cornea through the lens. These are larger in size. Sometimes, your doctor may prescribe 'piggy-back' lenses, i.e. a soft contact lens, which is large and sits snugly over the conical cornea and is comfortable, over which you wear a hard or RGP lens, to improve vision. There are special large lenses designed for Keratoconus, called "Rose-K2 lenses" after their inventor, Dr. Rose (nothing to do with the flower by the same name!).

The last option, which is horrendously expensive (around Rs. 90, 000/- for a single lens and Rs.1,40, 000/- for a pair, in 2010) is the Scleral Lens. The technical name for these is Scleral Lens Prosthetic Device or SLPD; the measurements for each patient are taken and the lenses are custom-made and dispensed. These lenses are very large, sit over the white portion of the eye, and are shaped somewhat like tea saucers. In the deepest part of the lens, a fluid is filled. The lens then sits on the eyeball, without touching the cone. The cone is always bathed in fluid, so there is both comfort and excellent vision. These lenses are long-lasting and do not need frequent replacements.

Q. What is the C3R procedure for Keratoconus?

A. You are remarkably well-informed. About a decade ago, in Germany, eye surgeons began experimenting with a procedure called "Collagen Cross linking of Cornea, using Riboflavin" (hence the term C3R...get it?) and a special ultraviolet light. The cornea is largely composed of fibres called collagen, which are interlinked with one other to give the cornea strength and allow it to retain its shape. In Kconus, the cross-linking between groups of collagen fibres is reduced, causing the cornea to stretch forward in response to the normal pressure from within the eye (intra-ocular pressure), thus worsening the cone. It was discovered that a combination of Ultraviolet-A light and Riboflavin (a component of Vit B-complex) could cause the collagen fibres to bond to each other more tightly, thus preventing the cone from progressing. The actual procedure is simple. Riboflavin drops are instilled onto the cornea surface, at intervals of every few minutes for 20 to 30 minutes, usually after scraping off the top layer, called the epithelium. Then, the ultraviolet rays are focussed onto the cornea, using a special lamp for about 30 minutes. The eye can be bandaged or a bandage contact lens inserted for a few days till the epithelium grows back. This procedure has a caveat however; the corneal thickness has to be a minimum of 400 microns, to prevent UV damage to the innermost layer of the cornea, the endothelium. Hence it cannot be done in advanced Kconus, where the cornea is already considerably thinned. The remarkable thing about this procedure, which has completed 5 years in patient treatment, is there have been hardly any cases showing progression of Kconus after the treatment and in some cases, there has been actual reversal with reduction in the spectacle number and astigmatism! Incidentally this procedure is also called CXL (short for collagen cross-linking)

Q. I do not wish to wear CL/cannot tolerate any CL/cannot afford the SLPD. My cornea is too thin to do C3R. Are there no surgical remedies? What about INTACS?

A. Yes, there are a host of surgical remedies. A few centres in India are using tiny plastic bands inserted into the periphery of the cornea, through a minor surgery. This causes the periphery of the cornea to stretch outward, thus flattening the cone. These plastic pieces are known as INTACS (Intra-stromal Corneal Segments). The upside is that it is a reversible procedure; the segments can always be removed. The downside is that it is not a very predictable procedure – one cannot estimate exactly how much correction will ensue, though there are some formulae which work as guidelines. The INTACS pieces are also currently not exactly cheap!

Q. Can we not do a corneal transplant?

A. We most certainly can. Corneal transplant or keratoplasty done for Kconus is very successful, with over 90% grafts remaining clear after 5 years. The traditional transplant is still penetrating keratoplasty or PK, where the entire thickness of the cornea (in the central 7-8mm zone), i.e. all its layers are transplanted or replaced by a similar or slightly larger disc of donor cornea which also contains all the layers. In India, this is how a vast majority of corneal transplants are done for Kconus.

However, increasingly, Indian eye surgeons are doing a procedure called DALK or deep anterior lamellar keratoplasty. The innermost layer or endothelium of the patient's cornea is quite healthy in Kconus and need not be sacrificed. Hence, in DALK, this layer is left behind. The donor cornea minus the donor corneal endothelium is transplanted. The procedure is technically a little more demanding. However, DALK leads to even less chances of graft rejection than PK and the recovery period is often reduced. Visual results are almost at par with PK.

For more details, please see the chapter on corneal transplants.

Nutrition and The Eye

This chapter is not written in the usual question-and-answer format of the rest of the book. No attempt has been made to make the chapter simple and easy to understand. It is meant to impress the reader that the author is actually capable of research (even if only on the Net and by going through various scientific journals). It is also meant to impress the reader with the author's command over complex technical jargon. The average reader may skip the chapter in its entirety. The above-average reader may however, read on.

I knew you would consider yourself above-average! Well then read on, but don't say I did not warn you!

Retinal diseases, including age-related macular degeneration (AMD or ARMD) are the leading causes of blindness in the developed world, while cataract is the leading cause of avoidable or preventable blindness in developing countries such as India. Epidemiological studies show that nutrition can play a role in the prevention and treatment of these potentially blinding conditions.

While proponents of alternative medicine believe that modifications in one's diet and nutritional supplements help to maintain healthy eyesight, most eye surgeons beg to differ. The truth lies somewhere in between. Let us examine the trends emerging from recent research and you can draw your own conclusions.

AMD

Age-related macular degeneration or AMD is an affection of the centre of the retina, called the macula. This region is responsible for all our near vision and most of our fine vision. Barely 20% of these cases, the so-called 'wet' types of AMD can be treated by laser. For the rest, there is no known cure.

Though the exact cause of AMD is not known, the macular area is rich in carotenoids such as lutein and zeaxanthin. Both contribute to the normal yellow appearance of the macula. Lower density of these pigments can increase the chances of light toxicity to the retina and macula. These act as scavengers of free radicals, which cause lipid peroxidation of the photoreceptor cell membranes, hastening the death of cells.

In 'wet' or neovascular AMD, persons with medium to high carotenoid levels have a significant lower risk of losing vision compared to those with low serum levels. One of the theories for why smokers are at increased risk of AMD is that smoking lowers serum carotenoid levels.

Vitamin E and AMD: Vitamin E, in the form of alpha-tocopherol protects one from AMD. In the Physician Health study that evaluated 21000 people over 12 years, it was found that 13.5% of the patients had reduced risk when Vitamin E supplements were given. This is however, not statistically significant. In experimental animal studies, chances of AMD increased if the subject was deficient in both Vitamin A and Vitamin E.

Vitamin C and AMD: When rats were given large doses of Vitamin C prior to prolonged light exposure, the macula seemed to be protected from light damage. Its protective action probably stems from its anti-oxidant properties.

Diet and AMD: In the Beaver Dam Study, 2000 people in the age group of 43-84 years were asked to answer a food questionnaire. It was discovered that the risk of AMD was inversely proportionate to the dietary intakes of carotenoids (fresh fruits and vegetables) and Vitamin E, a finding corroborated by several similar studies across the globe.

Spinach, collard greens, zucchini, green leafy vegetables (high lutein but low zeaxanthin content) and most fruits especially kiwi, grapes, oranges, yellow squash etc. are rich sources of carotenoids. Egg yolk and corn have highest levels of lutein and zeaxanthin (85% of total carotenoid content). Among vegetables, corn has the highest lutein content (60% of total carotenoids content) while orange pepper has the highest zeaxanthin content (37%). According to the Beaver Dam Study, moderate amounts of red wine, which is rich in flavonoids reduces the risk of AMD even if taken only once a month. On the other hand, beer increases the risk.

Zinc and AMD: Zinc is normally found in high concentrations in the retina, as it is required by several retinal enzyme systems. Low dietary intake of zinc increases the risk of AMD. An isolated report of a double blind study showed that zinc supplementation slowed the progress of AMD. In post-mortem examinations of retinas, those with AMD had decreased zinc compared to those without AMD.

Diabetic retinopathy

One of the causes of diabetic retinopathy (changes in the retina due to diabetes) is the development of glycosylated proteins i.e. attachment of sugar to proteins. These generate free radicals, which cause oxidative tissue damage and depletion of glutathione (GSH). These free radicals combine with lipids to form advanced glycated end-products (AGE), which damage blood vessels. Anti-oxidants block these processes and also reduce the permeability of capillaries (small blood vessels) in the retina.

Vitamin C, E and gingko biloba are anti-oxidants that prevent glycosylation. Magnesium and Vitamin B6 also help in slowing the progress of diabetic retinopathy.

Cataract

Cataract is the opacification of the lens of the eye. This occurs when the soluble proteins, which are in reduced form and therefore transparent are converted by oxidation to their insoluble oxidized form.

Glutathione levels in the lens decrease with age, resulting in faulty oxidative defence systems within the lens, thus causing cataract. Cataracts removed by surgery show a whopping 80% decline in glutathione (GSH) levels! This is due to decreased synthesis.

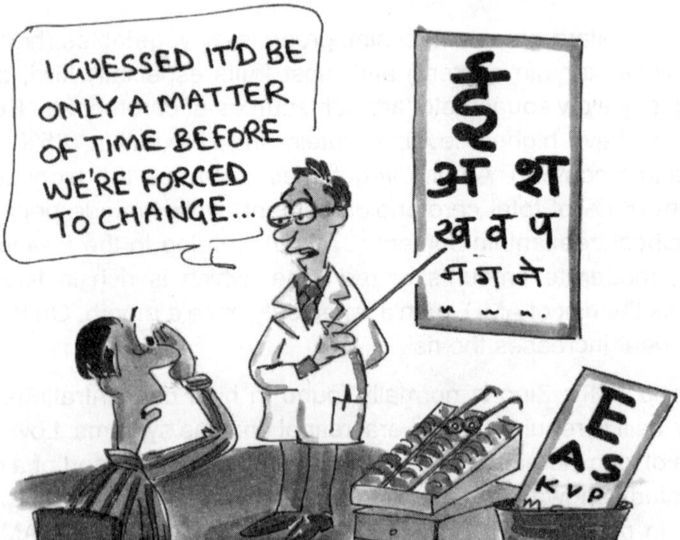
I GUESSED IT'D BE ONLY A MATTER OF TIME BEFORE WE'RE FORCED TO CHANGE...
E
A S
K V P
© Morparia

Cataract patients are also deficient in Vitamin A and the carotenoids, lutein and zeaxanthin. Smoking, ultraviolet B light, ionizing radiation, obesity, family history, oxidative stresses and several medications such as steroids, gout medications and heavy metals increase the risk of cataracts.

In the Nurses Health Study, over 50,000 women were given a food questionnaire. Those with higher consumption of lutein, zeaxanthin and Vitamin A had significantly fewer chances of developing a cataract. This is not true for beta-carotene, alpha-carotene or other carotenoids, however.

Vitamin E & cataract: Clinical studies have shown that low levels of Vitamin E increase the risk of cortical cataract. Rats given subcutaneous injections of 100 I.U. of alpha-tocopherol (Vitamin E) did not develop cataract when exposed to ionizing radiation unlike controls, who all developed cataracts. The same effect was noticed on substituting the injection with frequent eye drops of Vitamin E. In the longitudinal study of cataract, involving 764 participants, risk of cataract was 30% less in regular users of multivitamins and 57% less in regular users of supplemental Vitamin E. The conclusions of the study were:

- Vitamin E decreases oxidative stress in cataractous lens.
- Part of the Vitamin E effect is due to its ability to enhance glutathione levels.
- Vitamin E seems to protect against cortical rather than nuclear cataracts.

Vitamin C & cataract: In animal tests, steroid-induced cataracts in chick embryos were prevented by prior administration of high doses of Vitamin C. Cortisone decreases GSH levels; this process is slowed by Vitamin C. In the Nurses Health Study, supplementing the diet of 10-year-olds with Vitamin C led to 77% lower incidence of early lens opacities.

Riboflavin & cataract: In a trial involving 20,000 people in China, there was 44% drop in risk for persons taking a riboflavin/niacin combination. Riboflavin is a precursor of FAD, a co-enzyme for GSH reductase, which recycles GSH.

In conclusion, I would say, greater attention should be paid to nutrition in the management and prevention of potentially blinding eye diseases.

PTERYGIUM

Q. What is Pterygium?

A. "Pterygion" in Greek means "wing". Pterygium is a wing like growth from the conjunctiva (transparent membrane over the white of the eye), growing slowly over the cornea (transparent dome-like structure over the coloured portion of the eye). It is a degenerative condition that usually affects the nasal side of the eye i.e. the inner side rather than the outer side. It is usually harmless. As no one knows yet why pterygium affects some people and not others, it is believed to be genetic in nature.

Q. Who is at risk?

A. Pterygium affects people exposed to a lot of sunlight; hence those in the equatorial and tropical belts are more at risk. In USA, pterygium affects more people in sunny California than in cold and gloomy New York.

Q. Should all Pterygia be removed?

A. Never trouble trouble, till trouble troubles you. The same is true of Pterygia. Left to themselves, they are usually just a cosmetic blemish, growing very slowly over the cornea or not at all and compatible with good vision. However, if operated upon and removed using the modern technique of excision with conjunctival autograft, recurrence rates are 5-10% even in the best of hands. If the pterygium is simply excised and the exposed area on the sclera is not covered, the recurrence rates can be more than 50% at times.

Q. When should Pterygia be removed?

A. A pterygium should be removed if:

- It grows towards the centre of the cornea and encroaches on the papillary area,
- It grows rapidly,
- It causes symptoms, such as irritation, itching, etc.
- It interferes with the patient's vocation such as public performers, actors etc.

- It prevents the patient from wearing contact lenses.

In these cases, the benefits outweigh the risks of surgery. If a pterygium that has been operated upon recurs, it needs to be re-operated upon by an experienced eye surgeon.

Q. How is the Pterygium removed?

A. The technique, which is done for both primary and recurrent pterygia, was first described in 1985 by Kenyon et al. The pterygium which requires surgery is first excised very carefully. The size of the bare sclera is measured and accordingly, a free graft of the conjunctiva is taken from a normal section of the same eye. The graft is then sutured or glued into place. The donor area is left to heal on its own. A plastic conformer is placed in the eye for a few days to prevent adhesions to the raw surface. This method encourages good cosmesis and reduces the chance of recurrence.

Q. Can amniotic membrane also be used in this surgery?

A. Yes. Instead of using the patient's own conjunctiva, one can use amniotic membrane, a tissue available with the eye bank. However, the results are not as good as with the patient's own conjunctiva. The recurrence rates are a little higher with amniotic membrane – in one series, they were twice that of conjunctival autograft. However, if the patient has large Pterygia on both the inner and outer side of the eye or has had multiple recurrences, this may be the only option.

Q. Can those who have had successful Pterygium surgery donate their eyes after death?

A. Yes.

RETINA

Q. What is the "retina"?

A. The retina is the layer of the eye that is sensitive to light. It behaves somewhat like the film of a camera. It lines the inner surface of the back of the eye and is made up of several layers. Each cell of the innermost layer contributes a nerve fibre – millions of these nerve fibres join together to form the optic nerve.

Q. How do we see?

A. The front of the eye, chiefly the cornea and the lens focus the rays of light from any object onto the retina. Here, chemical reactions convert the light energy into electrical energy, which is transmitted by the optic nerve to the brain. This signal, coming from both eyes, is interpreted by the brain resulting in our perception of the object we are looking at. In other words, our eyes function like two TV cameras at a cricket stadium, with the brain acting as a master control room which fuses the two pictures sent by the two cameras into one, enabling us to see a single image and perceive depth as well.

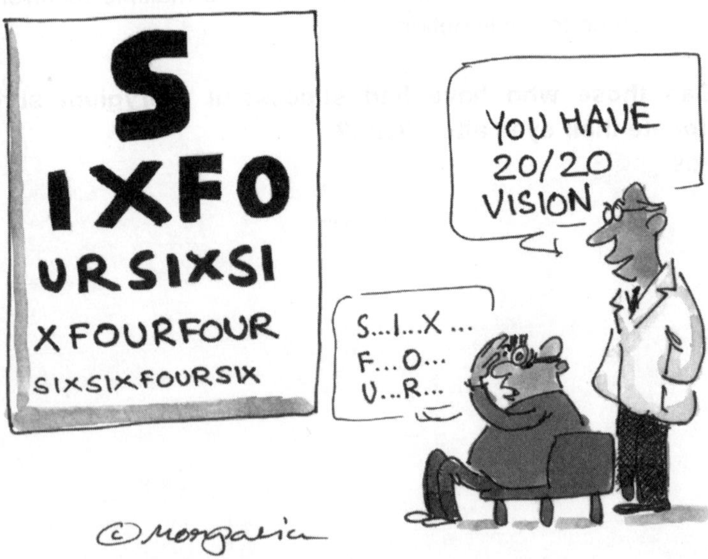

Q. I sometimes get pain in the back of my eyes. Is this due to some retinal problem?

A. No. The retina has no pain sensations. Whenever it is inflamed or stimulated it responds by giving you the sensation of a flash of light. Hence pain in the back of the eye is usually due to non-ocular causes such as sinusitis or some forms of migraine or tension headaches.

Q. I occasionally see flashes of light and some floating particles as well. Am I going blind?

A. Usually these are harmless. When you are 50 years of age, the jelly in front of the retina called the vitreous or vitreous humour may detach from its attachment to the retina. When this happens, there may be occasional flashes of light.

As you grow older, part of this jelly may liquefy with some of your own cells floating in it. When they float into your field of vision, you see them as black spots or 'floaters'. When they float out of your field of vision they may disappear from view. Sometimes, they may link up to form 'lines' or 'cobwebs'. If they do not increase in size or number, they can be ignored.

However, if there is a sudden increase in size or number of black spots or persistent flashes of light or if you are diabetic (see chapter on diabetes), hypertensive or shortsighted, it is better to consult your eye surgeon. He will dilate your pupils and examine the retina with an instrument called an 'ophthalmoscope' to rule out any serious cause for your symptoms.

Q. Can flashes of light or floaters indicate a serious problem?

A. Both these symptoms could indicate an early retinal tear or even a retinal detachment or vitreous haemorrhage. These are more common in diabetics, hypertensives and shortsighted people (those with minus numbered spectacles) and patients with bleeding disorders. Patients with these diseases should visit their eye surgeon for a retinal checkup at least once a year or more as advised by their eye surgeon.

Q. What is retinal tear or detachment?

A. A shortsighted person generally has a retina that is not proportionate to his slightly larger eyes. Imagine a fat person trying to wear the same shirt as a thin person. The shirt is naturally stretched and over time may get frayed or even tear. This is what happens to the retina in the eye of a shortsighted person. The stretched retina may give way at some peripheral area causing a retinal tear.

If there is a blood vessel just under the area which is tearing, it may tear too, causing leakage of blood or haemorrhage under the retina or through the tear into the jelly of the eye (vitreous haemorrhage). Initially, the floating blood cells or clots are seen as floaters. When the bleeding increases, it may obscure vision as well.

If the tear is not immediately detected and sealed, blood or fluid may seep through the tear and go under the retina, lifting it off its attachment to the underlying layer. This is known as a retinal detachment.

Q. How will I know that I may have a retinal detachment?

A. There is a chance of retinal detachment if you develop

- Sudden and persistent increase in the number of black spots in front of your eyes.
- Sudden and persistent increase in the flashes of light or decreasing duration between flashes.
- Sudden drop in quality or quantity of vision or cutout of a particular field of vision.

If you have the above symptoms, you should immediately rush to an eye surgeon.

Q. If I do have symptoms of retinal detachment, how soon should I consult the doctor?

A. Retinal detachment is an emergency. The earlier it is examined by an eye surgeon and operated upon, better the prognosis. If the surgery is delayed beyond a time, the detached retina may develop 'fixed folds', which make the retinal detachment surgery more difficult and time-consuming. It may involve additional procedures like vitrectomy to iron out those retinal creases or fixed folds from the inside. In spite of complex procedures, the retina may not settle in some cases. Longer the retina is left detached, less are the chances of a full visual recovery, even if the retina is successfully re-attached after the surgery.

Q. Is retinal detachment surgery very expensive?

A. First of all, seek an emergency appointment with the eye surgeon and let him confirm the diagnosis. He will discuss the surgical options with you at which point you can discuss your budget. Excellent retinal surgery is done at several trust and charitable hospitals, which will be well within your budget. Do not let the fear of raising funds prevent you from an initial consultation.

Q. What are the chances of success?

A. In a fresh detachment (one which is detected early) where the macula (the central light sensitive area of the retina) is not yet detached, the chances of anatomical success are close to 90%. The 'older' the detachment, more the fixed folds, higher the chances that the macula is also detached and lesser the chances of success. Each case is different – you should discuss the prognosis with your eye surgeon before surgery.

Q. What exactly is done in retinal detachment surgery?

A. First, the hole or tear in the retina responsible for the detachment is sealed either with a laser beam directed through the pupil or with a cryoprobe. The latter is a pencil like instrument applied to the sclera (white outer coat of the eye) just over the hole in the retina. The probe generates a very low temperature of -40°C to -70°C. This causes the formation of a temporary ice ball, which seals the hole or tear. The sclera is then pushed towards the detached retina with the help of rigid or soft silicon explants, encouraging the retina to come so close to its underlying coat that it will stick there permanently.

Q. When does a vitrectomy become necessary?

A. Vitrectomy is a procedure in which the vitreous (jelly of the eye in front of the retina) is removed and replaced by some heavy gases or silicon oil. It is performed during a retinal detachment surgery in the following conditions:

- ✦ If the retina does not settle after the first surgery, there may be some traction from the vitreous that causes it to remain detached.
- ✦ If the retinal detachment is accompanied by vitreous haemorrhage, preventing the surgeon from getting a clear view of the retina.
- ✦ If the surgeon sees traction bands in the vitreous which are responsible for the detachment. This is especially true in

diabetics who may suffer retinal detachment as a complication of their diabetic retinopathy.

- If the patient has an advanced cataract along with the retinal detachment, the surgeon may decide to remove the cataract as well as the vitreous to get a better view of the retina.
- If the patient has already had a cataract surgery but develops a thick 'after cataract' (thickening of the capsule at the back of the intra ocular lens implant) which precludes the view of the retina, the surgeon will excise the capsule along with the vitreous using the same vitrectomy cutter.
- If the retinal detachment has been caused by endophthalmitis i.e. an infection that has spread to the back of the eye, the vitreous is always removed as it is a hotbed for all sorts of germs.

Q. I am a shortsighted person, wearing minus numbered glasses. Should I give up reading or watching TV or sports to prevent retinal detachment?

A. Reading, studying or watching TV will not harm your eyes or make them more susceptible to retinal detachment. You can lift weights, swim, walk, jog or exercise as much as you like. Only remember to go for regular eye checkups as and when called. Rush to your eye doctor when your vision begins to fail suddenly or there is a sudden increase in black spots or persistence of flashes of light.

Q. My grandmother finds it increasingly difficult to read small print. She cannot recognise people even when they are close. She says though she can make out their outlines, their faces are a blur. She has already been successfully operated for cataract in both eyes. What could be wrong?

A. She probably suffers from age-related macular degeneration (ARMD or AMD) formerly called 'senile macular degeneration'. The macula is the most sensitive part of the retina. Located almost in the centre of the retina, it is responsible for fine vision and reading. Due to age-related changes, retinal cells become less efficient ('dry ARMD'), which may or may not result in mild scar formation at the macula. Sometimes, new, extra-leaky blood vessels may be formed below the macula, which may leak blood or fluid under the macula, causing a marked drop in vision ('wet ARMD').

Q. What are the early symptoms of ARMD?

A. In many cases, ARMD chiefly causes a gradual loss of central vision. If there is leakage of blood or fluid as in wet ARMD, this drop in vision may be sudden. The patient may complain of distorted vision - e.g. he will describe a window border as being crooked or bent. While reading, straight lines may appear crooked. Words may appear 'bunched up' or spread out. He may also fail to discriminate between colours properly.

Q. What is the treatment for dry ARMD?

A. For the dry type, there is no specific treatment. Anti-oxidant rich foods and anti-oxidant pills are supposed to delay the progress of ARMD, but the jury is still out on that one. There is no conclusive proof to indicate that these pills work. Many eye surgeons prescribe them nonetheless, as they feel 'at least, they do no harm' (except to the pocket of the patient)!

Q. What is the treatment for wet ARMD?

A. For the wet type, the eye surgeon usually conducts an FFA (fluorescein fundus angiography) test. A dye known as fluorescein is injected into a vein in the forearm. The dye reaches the retina in 10 seconds and then stains the blood vessels of the retina green. The patient is made to sit in front of a 'fundus' camera and serial pictures are taken at regular intervals. The eye surgeon examines the pictures looking for evidence of new blood vessels, site of leakage, distance of the leakage from the centre of the macula etc. Based on the findings, he may decide to apply laser to the retina at or near the macula.

There are several options in the laser treatment with argon laser or diode laser. The two new treatment options are:

- TTT or Transpupillary Thermo Therapy in which a modified diode laser gently heats the retina for about a minute.
- PDT or Photodynamic Therapy in which a dye called verteporfin is injected into a vein in the forearm. The dye settles in the new vessels under the macula. When laser light is applied, only the new vessels containing this dye are destroyed, leaving all other tissue undamaged. Unfortunately, only 10-15% of all macular degenerations can be subjected to any form of laser treatment.

Q. How can intravitreal injections of antiVEGF agents help in treating ARMD?

A. A lot of the damage in wet ARMD is caused by the abnormal proliferation of new vessels just under the retina. Vascular Endothelial Growth Factors (VEGF) promote the growth of new vessels in the body. If an anti-VEGF is injected into the vitreous close to the retina, it helps to prevent new vessels from sprouting and allows the existing vessels to close down.

Q. What anti-VEGF agents are available in India?

A. Currently there are three anti-VEGF agents in the market commonly known by their trade names – Avastin, Lucentis and Macugen. There are conflicting reports about which of these is better, so it would be wise to let your eye doctor decide which is best for you. Though Lucentis and Macugen are more expensive, they are approved by the US FDA for treatment of wet ARMD. Avastin is cheaper and is available in a multidose vial. But it is primarily an approved drug for treatment of colon cancer. It was found to be effective in the treatment of wet ARMD by chance! The treatment usually consists of a course of 3 injections with a gap of 4-6 weeks between injections. However, more injections may be required in some cases.

Q. Are there visual aids that can help my elderly grandmother to read large print?

A. There are special magnifiers called Low Vision Aids (LVA). Earlier, all we had were hand-held magnifying glasses. Now there are well equipped LVA clinics where you can get stand magnifiers, telescopic glasses and even use a computer to magnify the printed word and project it onto a TV or computer screen so that it appears many times its actual size.

Q. We are in the 21st century; can I not get a new retina to cure my grandmother's ARMD?

A. Experimentation with retinal transplants is going on in several centres around the world, including Hyderabad, India. However, this technology is in its infancy. It will still take several years before we can even know whether it will be at all effective in humans. At best, it may help patients who are blind in both eyes to see blurred forms with one eye.

Q. Can artificial retinal chips or miniature TV cameras help to restore sight?

A. They are being experimented with. After years of research, scientists have succeeded in making a bilaterally blind man appreciate the difference between light and dark. However, we are still several years away from affordable technology to help the average blind man see his loved ones.

Q. Can a person who has had retinal detachment surgery or ARMD donate his eyes after death?

A. Yes, provided his corneas are clear. It does not matter if the donor was blinded by retinal detachment or unsuccessful detachment surgery or if he had poor vision due to ARMD. As long as the cornea is clear, he can donate his eyes and restore sight to at least two persons suffering from corneal blindness. It is indeed wonderful that a person who was blind due to a retinal cause can help restore sight to two blind persons with opaque corneas!

SQUINT

Q. What is 'squint'? Is it hereditary?

A. Squint is an imbalance in the movement of the two eyes. Normally both eyes move in perfect harmony – when you want to look left, both eyes move effortlessly to the left side. Similarly, when you want to look straight ahead, both eyes will stay in the centre. If a person has a squint, one eye may not move at all in one direction (paralytic squint) or when one eye looks straight, the other may either diverge (move outward) or converge (move inward). Occasionally there may be a family history of squint – however most squints are due to spontaneous genetic factors and are not hereditary.

Q. What are the types of squint?

A. Squints may be either paralytic (due to muscle or nerve palsies) or non-paralytic. They are technically called non-concomitant and concomitant squints respectively. If the squinting eye diverges or moves outwards, it is a divergent squint. If it converges or moves inwards, it is a convergent squint.

Q. What is an "apparent" squint?

A. If the bridge of the nose is depressed i.e. the distance between the eyes is lesser or greater than normal, the child may have the appearance of a squint even if there is no real imbalance between the movements of the eyes. Most children grow out of this, though some may need plastic surgery to the face. However, it is best to let the eye surgeon decide which squint is real and which apparent.

Q. What are intermittent squints?

A. As the name suggests, these squints are not constant. They may be seen only when the child is day-dreaming, unwell, exhausted or emotionally upset. These squints are usually kept under observation. They may resolve spontaneously, thus requiring no treatment. If it becomes constant, treatment will be needed.

Q. Are all squints evident at birth?

A. No. Squints may be latent at birth and manifest after a few months or years. They may occur when the body's resistance is low e.g. after an illness. Certain squints may occur in adulthood, due to trauma or certain endocrine disorders like diabetes or thyroid disease or due to certain neurological conditions. A rare cause is iatrogenic, i.e. caused by eye surgeons mishandling the ocular muscles during eye surgery.

Q. If the squint is detected at birth, should I wait for my child to 'grow out' of it?

A. If the squint is divergent, it should be referred to the eye surgeon immediately on detection, as the only treatment for it is surgery. A divergent squint never resolves spontaneously.

If the squint is convergent, it should be referred before he is 3 years of age. Some squints are due to high hypermetropic refractive errors (accommodative squints) and can be corrected by appropriate plus powered spectacles and eye exercises.

Q. Should every child be referred to the eye surgeon by the age of 3 years to eliminate the possibility of a squint?

A. Yes. The ophthalmologist will look for refractive errors after dilating the pupil. The child's co-operation is not required. If necessary, corrective glasses can be prescribed to children as young as two years old. This can reduce or even eliminate an accommodative squint (see previous answer).

The ophthalmologist may also detect a marked difference between the spectacle numbers in each eye. If there is a number in only one eye there is a likelihood of the eye becoming lazy (amblyopic). The earlier this condition is detected, the better. The doctor will prescribe the correct number, patch the good eye and give stimulatory exercises to the lazy eye. This is best done before the age of 5 years. After the age of 8 years, chances of significant visual improvement are remote.

Q. Can any eye drops or Vitamin pills cure a squint?

A. There are absolutely no medicines for any manifest squint, except for those caused by endocrine or neurological disorders. Some intermittent and traumatic squints may resolve spontaneously over time.

Q. How soon should a squint be operated upon?

A. Divergent squints and convergent squints of the non-accommodative type (no significant refractive error) should be operated upon as soon as they are detected, as waiting does not help.

In the case of convergent squints caused by accommodation, corrective glasses are first prescribed and amblyopia treated if present. If the squint shows signs of improvement by these methods, surgery is delayed till there is no further improvement. The remaining or residual squint is then surgically corrected.

Q. Do squints cause psychological problems?

A. Yes. Children with obvious squints are often teased by their peers in school. They become shy, withdrawn and introverted. Even if they are bright, they refuse to interact in class and consequently often fare badly at studies. They develop an inferiority complex and may even become social misfits.

Q. Is squint surgery safe?

A. Yes. Modern anaesthesia ensures that squint surgery is safe even in newborns. There is no danger to the patient's vision, as the surgery is extra-ocular and the eyeball is not opened. Hence there is virtually no risk of blindness following squint surgery.

It is usually performed as a day care surgery under general anaesthesia. The bandage on the operated eye is removed after 24 hours. The stitches dissolve on their own leaving no scar. No special post-operative precautions or care are required. The child may have to apply drops for one month, but he can resume school in a week.

Q. Can squint be corrected at a later age?

A. Yes. Squints can be operated upon at any age for cosmetic reasons. In fact, many parents bring their unmarried daughters to correct their squints in the hope of improving their prospects in the marriage market! However, if the surgery is done after the child is 5 or 6 years old, the squinting eye is already lazy. Hence, even if the eyes are straightened by surgery, vision in the lazy eye cannot be restored. Therefore, squints should be ideally referred to an eye surgeon as soon as they are detected.

Q. Can squint be a marker for a serious eye disease?

A. Yes. An eye that is blind from birth or blinded later in early childhood due to unilateral cataract or eye tumour such as retinoblastoma or severe trauma can also develop squint. An eye surgeon will always rule out these disorders before he proceeds further with squint management.

Q. Can paralytic squints be corrected surgically?

A. Yes. Paralytic squints resulting either from birth trauma, such as forceps delivery causing 6th nerve or lateral rectus muscle paralysis or vehicular or other trauma in adulthood can be successfully corrected surgically using muscle tran-positioning techniques.

Q. To sum up...

A. Almost all squints can be corrected surgically for cosmetic purpose at any age. Best visual results are seen in patients whose squints are corrected in early childhood before the age of 5 years. If you know anybody with a squint, please advise him to visit an eye surgeon as soon as possible for an opinion – in case the squint is due to retinoblastoma, you may even save a life!

Q. Can people with squint donate their eyes after death?

A. Yes, they most certainly can. To donate eyes, all you need is a clear cornea, which almost all squint patients possess.

GLOSSARY

Angle: The cornea and the iris form an angle with each other called the anterior chamber angle or simply 'angle'. The Aqueous Humour flows out from the anterior chamber through the angle. If the angle is very narrow, there may be a hindrance to flow, causing the pressure in the AC to build up.

Anterior Chamber (AC): An optically empty space between the back of the cornea and the front of the iris. It is filled with a fluid called "Aqueous Humour".

Aqueous Humour: Made in a factory just behind the iris called the ciliary body. Flows forward from the posterior chamber, through the pupil into the anterior chamber.

Cataract: In old age, trauma, certain birth defects and certain diseases, the normally transparent lens turns opaque. This is termed cataract.

Choroid: A very vascular (filled with blood vessels) middle layer between the outer sclera and the inner retina.

Conjunctiva: A thin transparent membrane covering the sclera as well as the inner portion of both upper and lower eyelids. It stops at the junction of the cornea and sclera. In sore eyes, it gets inflamed, a condition called 'conjunctivitis'.

Cornea: The thin, multilayered tissue overlying the brown portion of the eye, similar to the glass in front of a wrist watch, except it is not flat, but dome shaped.

Fovea: A tiny spot within the macula which is the most sensitive area within the macula!

Glaucoma: If the pressure in the AC is greater than what the eye can safely bear without damage, the condition is termed glaucoma and the eye is termed 'glaucomatous'.

Iris: A flat, coloured circular tissue, which has an opening in its centre, the pupil, to allow light to reach the back of the eye. To carry the analogy of the wristwatch further, the iris lies where the face of the watch would be.

Keratoprosthesis: A synthetic or artificial cornea implanted in a patient who is unsuitable for a human corneal transplant.

Lens: Similar to the old film camera lens. It is slung like a hammock by tiny strands called ciliary processes which emerge from the ciliary body. Along with the cornea, it bends the rays of light to focus on the retina.

Limbus: The junctional area between the cornea and sclera. This is where the 'stem cells' are located, which replenish the outer, epithelial layer of the cornea.

Macula: A small area of the retina, which is most light sensitive, located very close to the exit of the optic nerve from the eye. Approximately 80% of details we see are due to the macula.

Ocular muscles: We have 6 eye muscles coming from the bony shell in which our eye is ensconced (the orbit) and attaching to the sclera. They are responsible for harmonious movement of our eyes in all directions.

Optic Nerve: Each retinal cell sends electrical energy via a nerve fibre to the brain. Approximately 2 million of these nerve fibres travel together in the 'optic nerve' taking the image to the brain, where they are interpreted by the higher centres.

Posterior Chamber: A narrow space between the lens of the eye and the back of the iris.

Posterior Compartment: Not to be confused with posterior chamber! It is a large 'empty' space between the lens and the retina. It is filled with an optically clear jelly called Vitreous Humour or vitreous gel or simply, 'vitreous'!

Pupil: The 'hole' in the centre of the iris. It expands from a normal of 2-3mm diameter to 6mm diameter when the person is excited. Does the same thing to allow more light to enter, when you are in a dark room. Functions like an adjustable diaphragmatic aperture of old film cameras.

Retina: A 10-layered structure at the back of the eye, like the film of a film camera. All light falling on it causes a chemical reaction. The energy released is converted into electrical energy.

Sclera: The tough white outer coat of the eye which protects four-fifths of the eye from damage. The front portion of the eye is protected by the transparent cornea.

Squint: An imbalance between the muscles of the two eyes.